that are
Killing you

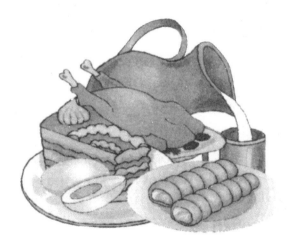

Foods That are Killings You

By
M. K. Gupta

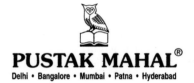

PUSTAK MAHAL®
Delhi • Bangalore • Mumbai • Patna • Hyderabad

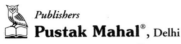

Publishers

Pustak Mahal®, Delhi

J-3/16 , Daryaganj, New Delhi-110002
☎ 23276539, 23272783, 23272784 • *Fax:* 011-23260518
E-mail: info@pustakmahal.com • *Website:* www.pustakmahal.com

Sales Centre

• 10-B, Netaji Subhash Marg, Daryaganj, New Delhi-110002
☎23268292, 23268293, 23279900 • *Fax:* 011-23280567
E-mail: rapidexdelhi@indiatimes.com
• Hind Pustak Bhawan
6686, Khari Baoli, Delhi-110006, ☎23944314, 23911979

Branch Offices

Bengaluru: ☎ 22234025
E-mail: pustak@airtelmail.in • pustak@sancharnet.in
Mumbai: ☎ 22010941
E-mail: rapidex@bom5.vsnl.net.in
Patna: ☎ 3294193 • *Telefax:* 0612-2302719
E-mail: rapidexptn@rediffmail.com
Hyderabad: *Telefax:* 040-24737290
E-mail: pustakmahalhyd@yahoo.co.in

© **Author**

ISBN 978-81-223-0007-9

7th Edition : August 2009

Printed at : Param Offsetters, Okhla, New Delhi-110020

PREFACE

There is a need of greater awareness about the foods we are eating. There are many foods which are silently killing us and compromising our health but we are hardly aware of it till we are stricken by an illness. We occasionally do hear about the harmful aspects of various foods but we don't pay much attention to these little warnings because of lack of awareness about their scientific aspect.

The purpose of this book is to increase your awareness about the harmful aspects of various foods by a proper scientific understanding and not by just repeating centuries old preachings of do's and don'ts, so as to have a better impact on the readers' minds.

I may also inform the readers that it is not necessary to accept blindly everything written in this book and in case of any doubt, they should also refer to other literature. It will be wrong on my part to claim that whatever I have written is final. I would also like to apologise to the readers for any discrepancies, if left inadvertently.

I am thankful to Mrs. Renu Singhal, Sr. Dietician, Safdarjung Hospital for having gone through the manuscript and for having given some useful comments.

With best wishes for the readers.

M.K. Gupta
Inter-University Accelerator Centre
(Formerly Nuclear Science Centre)
J.N.U. Campus, New Delhi-110067
Tel: 26892603, 26892601
E-mail: mkg@iuac.ernet.in

CONTENTS

White Sugar

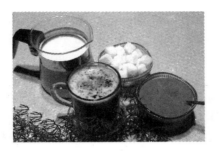

What is sugar

Sugar comes under the family of carbohydrates in our food. Before we discuss about sugar in detail, it will be worthwhile to have a brief knowledge about carbohydrates to have a better understanding about our main subject. Carbohydrates are basically compounds of carbon, hydrogen and oxygen. There are three types of carbohydrates in our foods.

1. **Monosaccharides:** They are also called '*Simple Sugars*'. This is the simplest form of carbohydrate and directly digestible in our system without any further breaking up into simpler compounds. Its chemical formula is $C_6H_{12}O_6$. There are three monosaccharides of importance in nutrition.

   i. Glucose

   ii. Fructose

   iii. Galactose

Glucose also known as *dextrose* or *grape sugar* is found in fruits, vegetables and honey.

Fructose is known as *fruit sugar* and occurs naturally in many fruits and berries. It constitutes over one third of sugar in honey and is responsible for its sweetness. These are major sweeteners used in carbonated beverages.

Galactose occurs as a component of a more complex carbohydrate in milk and the seed coat of legumes. It occurs in some fermented milk.

After the assimilation in the intestines, all these monosaccharides are finally converted by liver into glucose so that it is the glucose which finally goes to body cells for giving energy.

Simple sugars get into the blood stream very quickly after being swallowed. They need very little digestion and they don't have to undergo full digestive process. Some simple sugars can be absorbed right under the tongue.

2. **Disaccharides:** These are also called '*Compound Sugars*'. Disaccharides are made of two molecules of Monosaccharides. Its chemical formula is $C_{12}H_{22}O_{11}$. The most common disaccharides are

   i Sucrose   ii Lactose   iii Maltose

Sucrose is the most common disaccharide also known as *white sugar* or *cane sugar* which is the main focus of our topic. One molecule of sucrose consists of one molecule of Glucose and one molecule of Fructose. It is obtained from both sugarcanes and sugar beets. Sucrose is made up of one molecule of glucose and one molecule of fructose. What is available in market as 'Boora' and 'khand' also resemble white sugar in many respects. Hence they also have the same harmful effects on body as white sugar as explained later.

Lactose is known as *milk sugar* and it makes up half the total solids in the milk. It promotes the growth of micro organism 'Lactobacillus bifidus' known to be beneficial to young infants. One molecule of lactose consists of one molecule of Glucose and one molecule of Galactose. Lactose which is relatively insoluble is difficult to incorporate in solution and hence is not practical as a sweetening agent for liquids. However it is readily assimilable by the infant and has a laxative effect. It is less sweet than cane sugar while giving the same amount of calories. It consists of two simple sugars—glucose and galactose and is broken down in the small intestine by the enzyme "lactase".

Maltose also known as *malt sugar* is formed in malt (grain ferments) by the action of the enzyme *amylase* (present in saliva in mouth) on starch. One molecule of maltose consists of two molecules of Glucose. It is less sweet than cane sugar but it contains lime, iron and vitamins all of which are lacking in cane sugar. It is found in sprouting grains, malted wheat, barely and malt extract.

3. **Polysaccharides:** They are made of many molecules of monosaccharides with the molecular formula as $(C_6H_{10}O_5)n$. Following foods come in the category of Polysaccharides:

   i. Starch   ii. Cellulose

   iii. Dextrins   iv. Glycogen

Wheat, rice, maize, potatoes, peas, beans, millet are good sources of starch. We take these foods in the form of Roti (Chapati), Bread, Noodles, Rice, Dosa, Idli, Potatoitems etc.

Cellulose which comes from the cell walls of plants is also a carbohydrate but is not digested or absorbed by our body because our body doesn't have enzymes for digesting cellulose. When eaten, however, cellulose acts as a roughage or fibre and helps in keeping the intestinal tract in good working order.

Glycogen is stored in our body in the liver and muscles (by conversion of excess glucose into glycogen) and is utilised during periods of excess demand of energy by again getting converted into glucose.

Relative sweetening power of various sugars

Sugars differ in their sweetening power as shown in the following table indicating the relative values of different sugars considering value of sucrose or white sugar as 100:

Sucrose	100
Fructose	170
Glucose	70
Galactose	32
Saccharine	5500
Sorbitol	60
Lactose	30
Maltose	20

Note: (i) Saccharine is a synthetic sugar substitute and a coal tar product manufactured from toluene ($C_6H_5CH_3$). While pure, it has about 550 times the sweetening power of sugar but has no food or caloric value and may have harmful effects if used in excess, including its carcinogenic nature. While cane sugar stimulates the activity of the heart, saccharine depresses it.

(ii) Sorbitol is also a sugar substitute and is obtained from glucose through a chemical process in the form of alcohol sugar. It has less sweetening power and is less calorigenic than glucose. It is used in some weight reducing aids. It is found in many fruits such as peaches, pears and apples. It is used in chewing gums.

Requirement and role of sugar in body

Carbohydrates are the main source of energy in our body. However, all the carbohydrates can't be absorbed by our body as such. During the process of digestion, polysaccharides and disaccharides get broken down into monosaccharides or simple sugars which are absorbed by the blood. Liver converts all the monosaccharides into glucose which is then transported to body cells. Glucose is oxidised in the body cells to produce energy for carrying out body processes.

$$C_6H_{12}O_6 + 6O_2 \longrightarrow 6CO_2 + 6H_2O + \text{Energy}$$

Glucose　　　　Oxygen　　Carbon dioxide　Water

It may be noted here that it is not only the direct sugar eaten by us which adds sugar to blood but the starch etc., which initially may not appear sweet like sugar, also gets converted into sugar after digestion and adds to blood sugar in our body.

If the glucose or sugar in the blood is in excess of the immediate need of the body, then a part of glucose is converted into polysaccharide 'glycogen' which gets stored in liver and muscles. If it surpasses the body's capacity to store glycogen then the remaining glucose is converted into fat and stored in various parts of the body in the form of adipose tissues. In the case of excess demand of energy by body, these glycogen and fat get reconverted into glucose and supply the necessary energy.

As carbohydrates from ingested food is absorbed following a meal, the level of glucose in the blood usually rises and then falls gradually until it hits the fasting level resulting in onset of hunger. When the blood sugar level rises above 180 mg/ 100 ml, the condition is known as *hyperglycemia*. This occurs in *diabetes* where the lack of *insulin* (a hormone which controls blood sugar level) reduces the rate at which glucose is removed from the blood to the body cells for use as energy. Under these conditions blood glucose level gets so high that the kidneys, which normally reabsorb sugar to prevent its loss from the body, can't reabsorb the excess and sugar appears in the urine.

Blood glucose level below 70 mg/100 ml is known as *hypoglycemia*. This condition is followed by poor neuromuscular coordination, weakness, palpitation, sweating and eventually may lead to unconsciousness.

Brain is an important organ to be considered as far as glucose requirement is considered. Brain burns $2/3^{rd}$ of the body's glucose and it is highly dependent on the blood for a steady supply of this fuel, day and night. Its billions of electrical circuits are always turned on even when we are dreaming during sleep. Glucose generates 20-25 watt of electricity needed to conduct the brain's electrical business and also to produce the

13

neurotransmitters. Unlike muscles, brain doesn't have any store of glycogen of its own. So if you skip a meal or two and your blood sugar is running low, your body turns to its glycogen storehouse—liver, which contracts and supplies thedemand. Daily intake of sugar for a sedentary adult is expected to be around 20 gm (direct sugar excludin complexcarbohydrates).

So readers may note here that it is not that sugar is bad for the body. Body has a definite requirement of the sugar. But it is the quality and excess quantity of sugar which may produce harmful effects in the body. It is in this context that we shall study the harmful effects of *white sugar* or *sucrose*.

To inquisitive readers, I may also inform for their knowledge, that sugar also increases the entry of tryptophan (an amino acid) to the brain. There it produces 'serotonin' (a neurotransmitter) which is called a calming chemical and makes you feel good. This is perhaps the subsidiary advantage of sugar.

Harmful effects of white sugar

White sugar also known as *cane sugar* or *refined sugar* or *table sugar*, comes under the category of disaccharides and is chemically known as *sucrose*, as already described. White sugar is devoid of any vitamins, minerals or fibre because in the refining process all these things get removed. Hence it provides only empty calories due to which it has many harmful effects on the body as explained below:

1. White sugar robs the body of Vitamin B

Vitamin B (specially vit.B1 known as thiamine) is necessary for digestion and assimilation by the body of all carbohydrate foods - the sugars and starches. None of the B-vitamins are present in white sugar. Hence for assimilation and use of white sugar by the body, the B-vitamins are stolen from nerves, muscles, liver, kidneys, stomach, heart, skin, eyes, blood etc. This leaves these organs of the body deficient in

B-vitamins. Unless a large amount of food very rich in B-vitamins is taken, this deficiency will become worse and worse. As more sugar is taken, more B-vitamins are stolen. We thus suffer from nervous irritability, digestive disorders, tiredness, poor eyesight, anaemia, heart trouble, muscular diseases, skin diseases etc. It may safely be said that 90% of such troubles would disappear if use of white sugar is forbidden.

If you eat carbohydrates in natural form, you don't experience 'thiamine' (vit. B1) deficiency because thiamine to digest the sugar or starch is present in the food itself. Thiamine is required for growth, good appetite and smooth functioning of digestive tract.

2. White sugar affects heart

A definite relation of excess intake of white sugar to cardiac (heart) function has long been recognised. It impairs the functions of the heart. Thiamine deficiency caused due to white sugar causes a degeneration in the heart muscles and tendency to extravascular fluid collections and thus results in terminal cardiac standstill.

3. Sugar depletes energy

Thinking that sugar is energy, people eat more and more sugar in the belief that they are going to get more and more energy. But this is actually not true because of the two reasons - (i) the thiamine deficiency in sugar (and if other sources of vit. B1 are also lacking in the body) won't allow the completion of carbohydrate metabolism and energy fails to be released properly, and the result may be rather fatigue and less energy. (ii) Sugar high is often followed by a sugar low because of immediate rush of insulin when blood sugar level suddenly rises and this makes the sugar level below normal. The result is so called *hypoglycemia* attack in which symptoms of fatigue, dizziness, depression, tiredness, irritability, tremor and nausea may occur.

4. Sugar is a stimulant and increases sympathetic arousal

Sugar is a stimulant. A rise in blood sugar level immediately after eating sugar gives us a feeling of increased energy and leads to heightened arousal by increase in sympathetic activity. So after consuming white sugar, we may notice an increase in heart rate, a slight lift in blood pressure, increase in respiratory rate and infact in the entire tone of Autonomic Nervous System. Since all these changes in body's biochemistry are not accompanied by corresponding physical activity so as to dissipate this energy (which is being produced by increase in sympathetic tone) we feel stress. This is why sugar is often termed as 'stress food'.

5. Sugar causes calcium loss from the body leading to bone decay

Eating sugar changes the calcium/phosphorus ratio in the blood, with the calcium usually going up and phosphorus going down and therefore upsets homeostasis of the body. This calcium/phosphorus ratio remains disturbed for as long as 48 hours after the ingestion of sugar and therefore people remain out of homeostasis for a long time after eating sugar. Because of disturbance of this ratio, calcium is not fully absorbed by the body. Calcium and phosphorus work best in the ratio of 2.5 to 1. If calcium is more than 2.5 times the phosphorus, then extra calcium will not be absorbed or utilised by the body and will be excreted in urine or may form hard deposits in soft tissue. So you can be putting the right amount of calcium into your body, but when eaten with sugar, that calcium will not be absorbed efficiently. This is why the calcium of sweetened milk is never absorbed properly and may even induce a calcium deficiency disease called 'Rickets'.

In fact, sugar for its own metabolism and burning also requires calcium and since it itself is devoid of any minerals, this calcium is taken out of bones. This loss of calcium from the body will cause weakening of bones and teeth leading sometimes to 'osteoporosis'. Rickets, a calcium deficiency disease, can be attributed partly to intake of excess white sugar.

6. Excess sugar affects pancreas and causes diabetes

The eating of white sugar in large amounts may place a burden on the pancreas which secretes a hormone 'insulin' to enable the body to use sugar as fuel. Overworking of pancreas due to eating too much sugar will impair its functioning. Impaired or injured pancreas will lose the ability to secrete enough insulin thus causing the body to lose its ability to burn sugar. This condition eventually turns into the disease called 'Diabetes'.

7. Sugar causes tooth decay

Teeth get destroyed by excessive consumption of white sugar and sweets because sugar particles which get stuck in teeth, encourage the growth of certain bacteria which act upon the sugar and produce an acid which attacks the enamel of teeth. *Pyorrhea* - an inflammed condition of the gums (a form of arthritis) is caused by consumption of large quantities of sugar.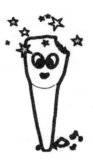

8. Sugar increases triglyceride level

Excess of sugar which can't be stored as glycogen in the body, gets converted into fat in the form of triglycerides and therefore leads to increase in blood triglycerides level, which can clog the arteries if present in excess and may affect the functioning of heart if coronary arteries are involved. Sugar also stimulates liver to produce more triglycerides endogenously.

9. Sugar undergoes fermentation

Sugars undergo no digestion in mouth and stomach. They are digested in the intestine. If taken alone, they are not held in the stomach for long but are quickly sent into the intestine. Sugars when eaten with other food, either protein or starches, are held up in the stomach for a prolonged period awaiting the digestion of other foods and undergo fermentation.

Sugars, as a law, ferment with all solid foods and milk. The fermentation of sugar leads to problems like acidity, gas, indigestion.

Note: Fermentation of sugar is the process in which it is broken down into alcohol and carbondioxide by the action of a fungus called 'yeast'.

10. Sugar increases acidity of blood

Sugar is an acidic food and increases acidity of blood which can lead to problems related to acidity.

11. Sugar increases constipation

Since sugar has no fibre, it increases the problem of constipation by not helping in bowel movements.

12. Sugar hinders starch digestion

By use of cane sugar in combination with various carbohydrates, salivary digestion gets bypassed. Saliva is an agent of supreme importance in the digestion of carbohydrate food and flow of saliva is normally aroused by mastication. By swallowing vast amount of sugar, the digestive action of saliva is missing and as a result, we must throw upon other digestive glands an abnormal strain which may affect their health.

13. Sugar increases uric acid

Sugar increases the amount of uric acid in the blood which can lead to gout and high blood pressure.

Common Eatables Containing White Sugar

1	Soft drinks
2	Sweets
3	Icecream
4	Canned fruit
5	Cakes
6	Pastries
7.	Cream roll

8	Tea, Coffee
9	Jams, Jelly
10	Toffees, Chocolate, Candy
11	Biscuits
12	Squashes (Sharbat)
13	Milkshakes, Icecream shakes
14	Sweet Lassi, Yoghurt
15	Sweetened milk and milk products

Better substitutes of sugar

1. **Sugarcane juice:** Although white sugar is made from sugarcanes only but the refining process removes many useful nutrients out of the sugarcane. Sugarcane juice contains vitamins B & C and is rich in organic salts of calcium, iron and manganese. It is recommended in anaemia and jaundice.

2. **Grapes:** Grapes which are good source of 'glucose' sugar, are equipped with vitamins A, B & C and minerals like calcium, phosphorous and iron.

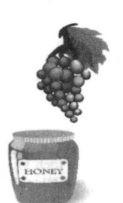

3. **Honey:** Honey contains nearly 75% sugar out of which 41% is fructose and 34% is glucose. It contains vitamins A, B (Thiamine, Riboflavine and Nicotinic acid) and Vit.C and trace minerals like Na, K, P, Cl, Fe. Honey provides following benefits to our body e.g.

   i. It strengthens the heart.

   ii. It is a natural and gentle laxative (cane or white sugar is constipative).

   iii. It is a blood purifier and is preventive against cold, cough and fever.

   iv. Honey is alkaline and doesn't produce acidosis or flatulence.

   v. Honey is a sedative. It is good for use in problems of 'insomnia'.

vi. Honey is a heart tonic and medicine for all ailments of the heart and blood pressure. Acetylcholine present in honey increases the blood flow to the heart and thus decreases the blood pressure and the heart rate.

4. **Molasses (शीरा):** It is the name of the liquid left after white sugar has been extracted from the cane or beet juice. Molasses (sheera) is a dark coloured syrup left after the crystallisation of sugar from the concentrated sugarcane juice. Molasses still contains about 30% of sugar which couldn't be separated by crystallisation. Sugar present in molasses is converted into ethanol (alcohol) by fermentation. Molasses is a by-product of sugar industry in India. Molasses has all the nutrient minerals and trace elements. It is also rich in vitamins B1, B2 and B6. An important constituent of molasses is phosphoric acid which is considered beneficial for brain and nerves. Molasses is good for stomach ulcers. It is good for the growth of breasts. It helps women during menopause. If taken during pregnancy, it ensures easy confinement and a healthy child. A teaspoon of molasses can be taken with a small cup of hot water.

5. **Jaggery (गुड़) and Brown Sugar (शक्कर):** These are made by heating sugarcane juice to a thick paste and then dried. They contain all the nutrient minerals and vitamins of sugarcane juice, since in making 'Gur' and 'Shakkar', molasses is not separated out and remains as a constituent part of 'Gur' and 'Shakkar'. They are specially rich in iron.

6. **Miscellaneous fruits:** It is better to fulfil sugar requirements from fruits like oranges, banana, carrots, beets, papaya, apple, mosambi, watermelon etc. The reason being that first of all they also contain necessary vitamins and minerals required for the metabolism of sugar. Secondly the sugar in them is in less concentrated form and hence doesn't increase blood sugar level so drastically.

Note: If fruits are made to over ripe, then the sugar changes either to acid or is fermented to alcohol by the action of micro organism 'yeast' which

Contd.

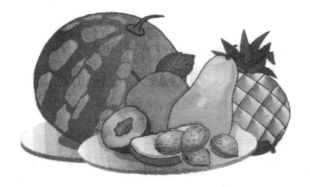

converts sugar of the fruit into alcohol and carbondioxide. Yeasts grow usually on food such as fruits which contain water and sugar. If fruits are eaten in underripe condition, then the sugar is still in the form of starch. During the ripening process, the starch gets converted into sugar.

7. **Complex Carbohydrates:** Try to take most carbohydrates in a complex form (i.e., starch etc.) because glucose resulting from the breakdown of starch is produced slowly as the starch is being digested. Pure sugar on the other hand rushes into the blood stream wholesale causing the blood glucose level to shoot up rapidly and creating a situation of 'sugar high'.

Further the sugars that are converted from the starches give the most sparing effect upon the vitamins manufactured in intestines. The reason is this: many vitamins are manufactured in the intestinal tract but to accomplish this, a friendly bacterial condition must be present in the intestine for the growth of bacteria which are responsible for the synthesis of vitamins. But the proper bacteria can't thrive without certain carbohydrate products and evidently these products result from carbohydrates such as starch that break down and absorb slowly. White sugar is rushed out of the digestive system too fast for the bacteria to work on them.

✿✿✿

Table Salt

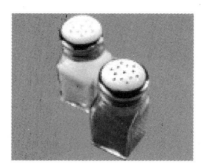

Introduction

The chemical name of the common salt is Sodium Chloride (NaCl). Sodium Chloride contains 39% of sodium, an element which never occurs in free form in nature. It is found associated with many minerals especially in plentiful amounts with chlorine.

Sodium chloride when dissolved in water yields sodium in the body and found in extracellular fluids. Sodium ions make up 93% of the basic ions in the blood. Common salt is obtained mainly from sea water. To recover common salt, sea water is run into lagoons and allowed to evaporate (A lagoon is a shallow salt water lake separated from the sea by sand banks). The sun's heat evaporates water and crude common salt is left behind.

Sodium chloride is highly soluble in water. When common salt is kept open, it absorbs moisture from the air due to the presence of small amount of magnesium chloride in it. Magnesium chloride ($MgCl_2$) is a deliquescent salt which absorbs moisture from the air to form a solution.

Requirement of salt in the body

Some amount of salt is definitely required by the body because of the following functions it serves in the body:

i. NaCl is an important constituent of our blood (0.9 gm in every 100 ml). It is important for the maintenance of Red Blood cells and helps proteins to dissolve.

ii. Sodium ions help in the conduction of nerve impulses and contraction of muscles.

iii. Sodium ions help to retain water in the body and maintain water balance.

iv. Sodium ions are important in transport of substances across cell membranes.

v. Sodium ions play a part in the electrical activity of the heart. Exchange of sodium and potassium ions in the pacemaker cells of the heart's sinoatrial node causes the heart to beat.

vi. Chloride ions are an important component of blood plasma.

vii. Chloride ions help in formation of HCl (Hydrochloric acid) in stomach for digestion.

viii. A saline drip is given to patients suffering from a severe loss of salts from the body as in cholera, dysentery, vomiting etc.

ix. Sodium plays an important role in the regulation of acid base balance in the body fluids including blood, lymph, tears and gastrointestinal secretions.

Experts suggest a maximum salt intake of 5 gm per day for an adult without a family history of blood pressure. If there is a family history then salt may be reduced to 2 gm per day.

However, increased salt intake is warranted during hot summer days and periods of heavy exertion that cause profuse sweating since salt and water are lost when we perspire or sweat. The white spots left on our coloured clothes by the drying sweat during summer are because of sodium chloride deposition. This is because when sweat dries from the clothes, water in it evaporates leaving behind sodium chloride which produces white spots on the clothes.

Severe salt loss in the body manifests muscle cramps, irritability and apathy.

Harmful effects of excess salt

i. **Salt is a stimulant:** It is stimulant. It stimulates Sympathetic Nervous System and adrenal glands and creates stress arousal. That's why it comes under the category of stress food.

ii. **High blood pressure:** Excessive salt causes water retention in the body and increases the blood volume and cardiac output resulting into High Blood Pressure. Considerable fall in B.P. is observed with reduction in dietary salt intake in Hypertension.

iii. **Weakening of bones:** Eating too much salt can pull calcium from the bones making them weak. More calcium is also excreted in the urine with the ingestion of more table salt.

iv. **Effect on Kidneys:** Excess salt puts a heavy burden on kidneys because they have to work harder to remove the excess salt. Hence they may gradually weaken. Kidneys can't remove more than 4-5 gm of salt per day. Remaining salt not able to be excreted gives rise to undesirable ailments in the body.

v. **Increase in weight:** Excess salt in the body increases the weight of the body because of the following reason. Kidneys eliminate excess salt from the body by filtering out the sodium that makes up part of the salt compound. In case kidneys work less efficiently either because they have gone weak or because of lowered blood supply to them (because of weak heart), the kidneys excrete sodium less efficiently and more sodium is retained in the body. Since the kidneys are

24

geared to maintain a fixed proportion of sodium to water in the blood, excess salt in the body means excess water too and hence excess weight of the body.

vi. **Worsening of Oedema:** Salt makes oedema worse and should be avoided in all edematous states whether due to liver, kidney or endocrine diseases.

vii. **Hardening of arteries:** Table salt is not completely soluble in water and tends to harden the arteries by its excessive use. For good health, that salt is required which is entirely soluble in water. High temperatures used for making table salt and elements like potassium chloride and sulphate and other chlorides tend to inhibit the dissolving of salt in water.

viii. **Salt increases uric acid:** Excess of salt interferes with the elimination of certain wastes of the system like uric acid and therefore contributes indirectly to various diseases like gout etc.

ix. **Bronchial and Lung problems:** Deficiency of organic sodium in table salt results in bronchial and lung problems because organic sodium is required for the elimination of CO_2 from the system.

Natural foods also contain salt

Actually speaking, there is some sodium salt present in every natural food we eat which is enough to meet the needs of the body under normal circumstances. Table below gives the sodium content of different natural foods.

Sodium Content of Different Foods
(mg. per 100 gram)

Food	Sodium content	Food	Sodium content
Onion	5	Wheat	18
Lemon	Nil	Bengal gram (Dal)	71
Drinking water	1-3	Tomato	46
Lentil (Whole)	40	Pumpkin	6
Potato	11	Cashewnut	Nil

Contd.

25

Food	Sodium content	Food	Sodium content
Carrot	36	Groundnut	Nil
Spinach	58	Radish	33
Cabbage	Nil	Brinjal	3
Guava	6	Banana	37
Grape	Nil	Milk (Buffalo)	19
Green gram (Whole Moong)	28	Egg	129
Bajra	10	Mutton (Muscle)	33
Cucumber	10	Peas (green)	8
Apple	28	Fenugreek	76

Hence one has to calculate his sodium intake taking into account the above sodium contents present in natural foods.

Common eatables (processed/ cooked foods) containing table salt

We are consuming table salt in various processed foods (in addition to salt consumed from natural foods as described earlier) such as (i) soft drinks (ii) sauce, ketchups (iii) cornflakes (iv) salted biscuits (v) processed cheese (vi) butter milk,  lassi (Namkeen), (vii) raita (viii) salad with salt sprinkled over it (ix) pickles (x) tinned and canned vegetables/fruits (xi) papads (xii) potato chips (xiii) roasted badam, cashewnuts, peanuts (xiv) pasta (xv) cooked vegetables and dals (xvi) sandwiches, pizzas (xvii) chinese foods (xviii) chutney (xix) soup (xx) pakoras, patties, samosas (xxi) salted butter.

Please also remember that there are other forms of sodium also than those found in table salt. Sodium nitrate is used to preserve many processed foods. Scientists have discovered that sodium nitrate can cause cancerous tumours if ingested over a period of years. Another way to obtain sodium is through monosodium glutamate commonly known as MSG. It is commonly found in Chinese foods as well as canned, frozen and packaged foods. MSG is used to enhance flavour. Although it tastes less salty than table salt, it has three times the sodium content.

Recommendations/better substitutes for table salt

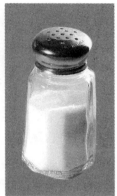

i. Table salt is an inorganic material and a strongly ionic bonded material and resists being separated into the sodium and chloride ions that are usable by body. Hence it doesn't replenish properly the sodium needed for our body. While the salt in fruits and vegetables is organic in nature and loosely covalently bonded and can be easily utilised by body. Hence we should try to reduce the intake of table salt and suffice our requirement by intake of natural foods. Infact whatever amount of salt is needed by body is already provided by the natural foods we take daily.

ii. Rock salt is considered better than table salt. Rock salt deposits are found in some mountainous regions. Salt is dug out from the rock salt deposits. It exists dissolved in water if found very deep. The saturated solution is then pumped out and evaporated to get the salt. Rock salt has been found to be entirely soluble in water and the body enzymes can make good use of it thereof.

iii. Black salt (Kala Namak) is also considered better than ordinary table salt because it (black salt) is organic in nature.

iv. For High B.P. patients, potassium salt is recommended than sodium salt. Such salts are now a days available in the market with the brand names 'Annapurna salt', 'Lona salt' (ayurvedic), 'Saffola salt' etc.

✿✿✿

27

Coffee and Tea

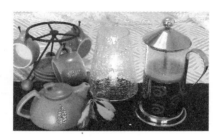

Introduction

Drinking some type of caffeinated drink is a part of our culture and every day life. We visit a friend and the first thing we find is a cup of tea or coffee.

Today the coffee pot is an indispensable fixture in most offices. Business meetings break for coffee and in every corridor in every organisation is a sophisticated coffee and tea making machine. A cup or two of coffee seems to give the burst of energy sought by office workers each morning as well as by long distance drivers through the night. And in your own life, you may find yourself drinking a caffeinated beverage to gain a slight edge on a mental task such as holding a meeting, writing a letter, doing some calculation. It is caffeine contained in all these drinks which really plays havoc with your body and mind.

Coffee is obtained from the seeds of an evergreen plant. Seeds of the fruits of this tree are roasted and ground. This is the coffee powder sold in the market.

Mechanism of action

The chemical name of caffeine is 1,3,7-trimethylxanthine. In its pure form it is a bitter tasting fine white powder looking rather like icing sugar. It is soluble in water and so is easily absorbed into the blood stream and rapidly reaches the brain where its most remarkable effects are felt. In general, a single dose of caffeine will appear in the bloodstream within 10 minutes of drinking it. It then reaches a peak concentration between 30 and 60 minutes after taking it but absorption is much slower when the stomach is full.

Experiments which measured the electrical activity of the brain have shown that the caffeine in just one or two cups of instant coffee dramatically changes the pattern of brain activity from a typical resting state to that of an alert, very awake person. That's why caffeine has been termed as 'Psychoactive Drug'.

Caffeine has its effect on the brain by blocking the action of 'adenosine', another psychoactive chemical found throughout the body. Adenosine slows down the release of neurotransmitters - chemicals that carry messages from one nerve cell to another. It has a calming effect on body. Without the calming and controlling effect of adenosine, nerve cells continue to fire and fire more rapidly. Caffeine blocks the action of adenosine and thereby keeps one stimulated.

Caffeine also stimulates the adrenal glands to raise the level of stress hormones - adrenalin, nonadrenalin and cortisol. These are the ones that are released when we are anxious, scared, angry or nervous and produce the 'fight or flight' response. These hormones energise and stimulate the brain. Hence overall, caffeine not only increases the body's stress levels (by release of stress hormones) but also blocks the action of 'adenosine', one of the body's de-stressing chemicals. No wonder we feel high and alert after every cup of coffee.

Duration of effect of caffeine

Caffeine will continue to have its effects as long as it remains in the bloodstream. In the meantime, enzymes in the liver work to breakdown the drug and remove it from the system. The half life of caffeine - the amount of time it takes for the liver to metabolise half of the amount that has been taken in, varies a great deal between individuals. The usual half life for an adult is between two to ten hours, with an average of around four hours. This huge variation explains why some people can drink large amounts of coffee without much effect while others feel jittery, anxious and simply can't tolerate caffeine. Men and women tend to have similar rates of caffeine metabolism.

Smoking stimulates the enzymes that metabolise caffeine and smokers have a 50% faster rate compared with nonsmokers. This means that smokers experience the effects of caffeine for a shorter time and possibly drink more to compensate. Other drugs such as alcohol reduce the rate of caffeine breakdown and the oral contraceptive pill can triple the half life of caffeine. Thus women on the pill tend to react strongly to a second dose of caffeine because there is still a large amount waiting to be metabolised.

Tolerance to caffeine

People who drink a lot of coffee on a regular basis do develop a tolerance to it, meaning they need to drink more to get the same effect. In fact, once you get to this level, caffeine starts to have other less desirable effects on the body. In a sense you become over stimulated; you are jittery, anxious, nervous, unsteady, on the edge all the time as caffeine disrupts the fine motor coordination within the nerves. These are also the symptoms that drive people to their first cup of the day.

Addiction to caffeine

Caffeine is a habit forming and addictive substance although it is not technically classified as an addictive drug as every body doesn't become a slave to it. But certainly many people depend on it and suffer significant withdrawal symptoms. This is because as the initial stimulating effect of caffeine wears out, the person craves for another cup to experience the same lift. People taking more than 4 cups a day become normally dependent on it and are likely to suffer damaging withdrawal symptoms.

Many withdrawal symptoms are experienced by person who is hooked to caffeine and misses its regular consumption for some reason e.g.

1. One will experience a withdrawal headache approx. 18 hours after his last cup of coffee or tea. The pain is likely to become more intense for 3 to 6 hours and may persist for a day or longer.

2. One has the feeling of dizziness when he first stands up after lying down because of lack of blood flow to the brain of caffeine victim.

3. Morning fatigue and tiredness: person doesn't feel energy in the morning even though he has slept the proper amount the night before. He gets tired in the late afternoon and has to nap.

4. Diminished concentration and mental fogginess.

5. Anxiety, anger, depression.

These symptoms are often relieved by rushing again to the cup of coffee but it only creates a vicious circle reinforcing the addictive habit further.

Caffeine Containing Drinks and Foods

	Average amount per 150 ml cup or as stated (mg)	Range (mg)
Ground Coffee	115	60-180
Instant Coffee	65	30-120
Tea	40	20-60
Cocoa	4	2-20
Drinking Chocolate	4	2-15
Cola drinks (330 ml can)	40	30-40
Dark Chocolate	80	70-90
Milk Chocolate	20	4-60
Painkillers (2 tablets)	60	30-130

Note: (1) The range is given mainly because of wide variation in the quantity and quality of the coffee and the size of cup etc. (2) Dark chocolate contains 4 times as much caffeine as milk chocolate.

(3) The amount of chocolate in a serving of ice cream or pudding is negligible in terms of the amount of caffeine it provides.

Temporary benefits of caffeine

1. Caffeine has been found to substantially increase wakefulness and clarity of mind. Thoughts may come more easily for a while, decision time may be shortened and some people find they can focus their attention better.

2. Initial boost or lift given by caffeine temporarily staves off fatigue and inertia.

3. A hot cup of coffee, as a first aid, relieves asthma because caffeine dilates bronchial tubes.

4. Some people find they can chase away a minor headache with a cup of coffee. In fact many over the counter cold and headache pills contain caffeine.

But all these benefits are of temporary nature.

Harmful effects of caffeine

1. **It drains energy:** Although intake of caffeine gives an initial boost or lift to the mind, but soon it is followed by a let down and you feel more drained of energy. Symptoms of fatigue, tiredness and irritability are often found in caffeine addicts.

2. **It increases urine output:** Caffeine is diuretic and increases the urine output.

3. **It causes calcium loss:** Caffeine administration increases faecal and urinary calcium excretion resulting in calcium deficiency and also the deficiency of other minerals, e.g. sodium, magnesium and potassium, etc. Calcium loss may be greatest when caffeine is taken with sugar.

4. **It raises cholesterol:** Boiled coffee contains a lipid that powerfully raises serum cholesterol. HDL cholesterol remains unchanged. 4 cups of coffee can increase cholesterol in the blood by 5% and ten cups by around 12%.

5. **It hinders assimilation of food in intestines:** With the use of caffeine, the inner side of intestines gets coated

and stained that hinders the proper participation of the intestines in the digestive process. Other digestive tract problems such as colitis and piles can also be aggravated by caffeine.

6. **Harm to breast-fed infant:** In quantities of more than 200 mg in a day, caffeine can be passed through the breast milk to the nursing infant. Caffeine intake during pregnancy may lead to maternal and infant anaemia.

7. **Loss of vitamin B:** B vitamins are lost when a lot of caffeine is taken. These vitamins play a crucial role in energy metabolism and so with a high caffeine intake, the body is losing the very nutrients that are needed to produce energy. No wonder we feel tired both in mind and body.

8. **Effect on Heart:** Caffeine causes increased and irregular heart beat (arrhythmia) and increases blood pressure. This can lead to increased workload for heart and can be a danger for those with coronary heart disease.

9. **It increases acidity:** Caffeine stimulates the production of acid in the stomach. This can cause heartburn, indigestion and aggravate ulcers. These problems become much acute if coffee is taken in stressful state of mind because during stress response stomach reduces its emptying time and coffee at this time will stay in the stomach longer and have more time to exert its harmful effects. That's why persons having problems of acidity should reduce their intake of coffee and tea and persons having ulcer had better avoid them completely.

10. **Sleep disturbance:** Caffeine alters normal sleep patterns. Caffeine users are more easily aroused by sudden noises and they are generally a lot less settled during sleep and don't feel fresh after waking up. It is thought that caffeine affects the quality of REM sleep (dreaming sleep). Without adequate REM sleep we become fretful, irritable, tense and less able to concentrate.

11. **Headache, irritability, anxiety:** Caffeine victims often complain of headache as an after effect and

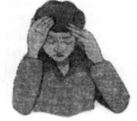

generally show irritability, anxiety, depression. Infact coffee & tea have been listed among Migraine triggers.

12. **Effect on Kidneys and Liver:** Since kidneys and liver have to overwork in the body of caffeine victim, so these may suffer after sometime. This is why people with kidney and liver disorders are advised to refrain from coffee and tea.

13. **It raises blood sugar and aggravates diabetes:** Since caffeine raises the blood sugar level, so it can aggravate the existing diabetes problem.

A few words about tea

Although both tea and coffee contain caffeine, the concentration of caffeine in tea is much less and tea also has some other redeeming qualities such as

1. 'Tannins' in tea destroy bacteria and virus and therefore it inhibits the growth of dental plaque. But at the same time 'tannin' is also implicated in inhibiting the absorption of iron, calcium and zinc from food when tea is consumed at meal times. Tannin is also said to stain teeth.

2. Tea is rich in flouride. This helps the teeth in avoiding cavities.

3. Tea is a potent mouthwash and good for gargling.

4. Tea has antioxidant power to neutralise free radicals because it supplies an antioxidant 'quercetin'. Thus it lowers the risk of heart disease and cancer to same extent.

   Hence tea can be occasionally taken in moderation but remember, that it has all the disadvantages of caffeine.

Better substitutes for coffee and tea

1. Use decaffeinated tea and coffee. In these drinks, caffeine is removed from the coffee beans or tea leaves at the green stage with water or a solvent.

2. Green tea is better than black tea. Green tea is said to reduce blood pressure, strengthen blood vessels, prevent thrombosis and treat infection.

3. Herbal tea and lemon honey tea are considered a good substitute for black tea.

✿✿✿

Smoking and Tobacco

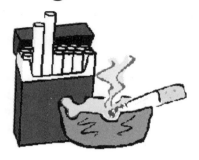

Smoking as addiction

If you use cigarettes to calm you down when you feel stressed; if you don't feel at ease in the morning until you have lit up; if you feel tense and irritable and have headaches if you can't smoke and find it difficult to concentrate without smoking, then you are addicted to smoking. What hooks smokers or makes them addicted? Studies suggest that they are addicted to nicotine's effects on the brain. Nicotine gives a temporary lift to the smoker. But soon it is followed by a let down and smoker craves for another bout of smoke to experience the same lift again. This is how nicotine creates addiction. Gradually over a period of time, when one becomes addicted, smoking is also continued to avoid withdrawal symptoms such as anger, anxiety, difficulty in concentrating, hunger, impatience, restlessness and cigarette thus establishes itself as an integral part in one's daily life.

Nicotine is metabolised fairly rapidly, disappearing from the body in a few hours, so smokers have to take frequent puffs in a day to maintain the lift. A typical addict smokes between 10 and 50 cigarettes each day. Nicotine can be ingested through other ways also e.g., Pan chewing or eating tobacco directly.

How Nicotine reaches the brain

Smoking creates a fast track to the brain. When you puff on a cigarette, every breath fills the air sacs in the lungs with a fresh supply of nicotine which passes into the blood before that breath is exhaled. A meshwork of fine capillaries surround each tiny air sac, enabling all the blood in the body to pass through the lungs - about five litres every minute. From the lung, all the blood goes to the left side of the heart. From there, as it is pumped out, a certain portion goes to the brain. Hence the brain is swamped by a new inrush of nicotine immediately after inhalation. Nicotine reaches the smoker's brain even faster than if it had been injected into a vein - within just six to eight seconds after inhalation, giving the smoker near immediate effect.

Because nicotine reaches the brain in small spurts, the smoker is able to control the rate of intake. For more effect, smokers take deeper or more frequent puffs. If a toxic concentration in the brain is being approached, the smoker feels dizzy or nauseated and stops smoking or slows down.

Effect of Nicotine on Brain and Mind

Nicotine works by stimulating the release of neurotransmitters and neurohormones in the brain. Light a cigarette or take a chew or dip some snuff and you are tampering with your brain's chemistry.

At low doses, nicotine stimulates the release of *beta-endorphin*, an opiate made by the body. Consequently smokers feel calmer. In contrast, high dose prompts the release of *nonadrenaline*, *adrenaline* and *dopamine*. Smokers may experience a lift or find themselves in the paradoxical state of being both more alert and relaxed. It is understood that these neurotransmitters/hormones stimulate the pleasure centre of the brain which keeps the smokers addicted to smoking. Nicotine has also been credited with improvements in mental performance through an increased release of two neurotransmitters involved with memory function - *Acetylcholine* and *Vasopressin*.

However these brain stimulating effects don't last for long—from 15 minutes to half an hour and these benefits are temporary only, while the harms caused are much more as explained later.

Harmful effects of smoking

In the cigarette smoke, over 400 chemicals have been found to be hazardous to health. A light smoker consuming only half a packet a day bombards his body with these chemicals about 3500 times a year. However, three most harmful substances in cigarette are—

a. **Tar:** It is a carcinogenic (cancer producing) substance.

b. **Nicotine:** Nicotine is a poisonous substance that has long been used as an insecticide and rat poison. It is considered only second to the cyanides in its destructive effect on human body.

c. **Carbonmonoxide:** It is the gas present in cigarette smoke.

Various harms done by the harmful substances in the cigarette smoke can be summarised as follows:

1. **Irritation of mucous membranes of the lung airways:** The substances contained in smoke are transferred to the bronchial tubes and the lungs and are deposited on the mucous membranes (lining these tubes) where they cause much local irritation. In fact these mucous membranes may become four or five times thicker in the heavy smoker than in a non smoker. This increases the resistance to the passage of air into the lungs and makes it that much harder for him to breath.

2. **Peptic Ulcer:** Smoking significantly increases secretion of acid in the stomach and leads to stomach ulcer.

3. **Respiratory Illnesses:** Smokers have continuous trouble with their throat and lungs, having chronic hacking bronchitis and stubborn coughing, finally leading to severe

breathlessness because of gradual destruction of lungs as explained in point no. 7.

Atmospheric pollution has an additive effect in smoker's problems. Smokers can have frequent pneumonias and asthmatics find their disease further worsening.

4. **Osteoporosis (Weakening of bones):** In smoke is found a heavy metal called cadmium which can cause extensive bone loss. Even extremely low levels of cadmium (similar to those in women who smoke) can result in 30% loss of bone calcium.

    In women, cigarette smoking has been shown to stop estrogen activity and anything that stops estrogen from functioning is likely to cause osteoporosis. This may lead to frequent bone pains and occurrence of spontaneous fractures.

5. **Earlier Menopause:** Women who smoke reach menopause an average of five years earlier than non smokers.

6. **Effect on pregnant women:** Pregnant women who smoke, run the higher risk of incurring abortions and foetal deaths. Their newborns can have sudden deaths. The long term intellectual growth of babies of smoking mothers can get affected. Concomitant use of oral contraceptives such as mala-D by smoking women can lead to heart attacks and strokes.

    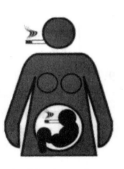

7. **Damage to Alveoli of lungs (Emphysema):** Noxious fumes of smoking damage the lining of many tiny alveoli in lungs. This tremendously reduces the surface area in which oxygen comes into contact with blood and results in a condition called 'Emphysema'. It develops slowly and silently over a period of time. All smokers have 'emphysema' to some degree but because of the enormous area that exists for diffusion of O_2, most people are not aware that they have this condition (Most people have about 300 million alveoli in their lungs). It is only when this area becomes drastically reduced that

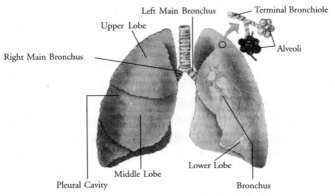

Left Main Bronchus
Terminal Bronchiole
Upper Lobe
Right Main Bronchus
Alveoli
Middle Lobe
Lower Lobe
Pleural Cavity
Bronchus

Smoking damages the Alveoli of the lungs

one finds he can't exchange enough gas to keep up with his oxygen needs. He will notice this during exercise, for example, and feel short of breath.

8. **Reduction in oxygen carrying capacity of the blood:** Carbon monoxide (CO) is present in high concentration in smoke. The affinity of the CO for Haemoglobin is 200 times greater than that of oxygen. Hence some of the haemoglobin of the blood remains tied up with CO in smokers and oxygen carrying capacity of the blood is remarkably reduced.

9. **Cancer:** Over forty eight cancer initiating, cancer promoting and cancer accelerating agents known as carcinogens have been identified in cigarette smoke (e.g., aromatic amines, nitroseamines, aromatic hydrocarbons, catechol etc.). Lung cancer is the most common among smokers. If your occupation involves activities like mining or exposure to asbestos, the risk multiplies manifold. Many other cancers like cancer of the throat (the voice box), mouth cancer, cancer of the food pipe (oesophagus) and of the urinary bladder are also commonly seen in smokers. Cancers of the kidney, pancreas, stomach and the cervix have also been occasionally noticed in smokers.

10. **Loss of vitamins:** Smoking has an adverse effect on the vitamin stores of the body, specially vitamin C. It has been noticed that taking just one cigarette consumes

39

vitamin C of the body equivalent to contained in one orange. Hence smokers need lot of intake of vitamin C for compensating the loss.

11. **Effect on Heart and Cardiovascular system:** In three different ways, cigarette smoking can affect one's cardiovascular system.

   a. Nicotine stimulates sharp release of stress hormones—adrenalin and nonadrenaline (also called epinephrine and nonepinephrine) which increases heart rate and blood pressure. It leads to more demand of oxygen by heart muscle whereas CO (carbon monoxide contained in smoke), on the other hand, decreases oxygen carrying capacity of blood. Smoking thus causes heart to overwork without any outward requirement which eventually weakens the heart and leads to palpitation. In an experiment, it was found that smoking just two cigarettes caused a blood pressure rise of 8-10 mm which then stayed high for 15 minutes or more.

   b. Smoking increases blood viscosity as well as clot formation and therefore, aids atherosclerosis and thrombosis. Coronary arteries and arteries leading to the brain are most affected in this phenomena.

   c. Smoking damages platelets in blood.

   d. Smoking increases LDL cholesterol (harmful cholesterol) and decreases HDL cholesterol (good cholesterol) and leads to hardening of arteries. Two factors in smoking are said to be responsible for these things:

      i. Carbon monoxide in the blood contributes to hardening of arteries and makes its lining rough which encourages cholesterol deposition.

      ii. Lack of Vit.C due to smoking causes the deposition of cholesterol in the arteries.

12. **Stroke and Paralysis:** Since smoking increases blood viscosity and clot formation, the occurrence of stroke or a paralytic attack is commoner in a smoker than a nonsmoker.

13. **Smoking increases blood sugar level and causes diabetes:** Nicotine boosts blood sugar by stimulating the flow of adrenaline and nonadrenaline which in turn causes the liver and muscles to discharge glucose into blood stream. This puts pressure on pancreas which has to secrete insulin again and again to control the blood sugar and can get eventually weakened by overwork leading to diabetes.

14. The gas phase of cigarette smoke contains nitric oxide and nitric dioxide both of which can be termed free radicals as they carry an unpaired electron and are capable of initiating free radical chain reactions. For details of damage to body by free radicals please refer chapter 8.

Quitting smoking

Here are some tips to help you to quit smoking:

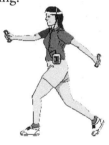

1. One of the best helps in quitting smoking can be provided by regular aerobic exercise. This is a habit that like smoking increases the release of beta-endorphin, acetylcholine and adrenaline. The result of a good aerobic workout is that same paradoxical state of relaxed alertness. And unlike smoking, there are no health hazards also.

2. Take help of nicotine replacement therapies such as nicotine gum, patches, nasal spray and inhalers as well as non-nicotine medicines such as bupropion.

3. Set a special date for quitting smoking such as your birthday or your anniversary. Psychologically you can gather more mind power on these days for quitting smoking.

4. Don't do mechanised smoking. Be aware whenever you start smoking. This awareness will help you in quitting smoking because smoking is always done unconsciously.

5. Increase intake of those foods which make smoking incompatible with them, e.g. milk, fruit juice instead of tea, coffee.

6. Stop carrying cigarettes with you at home and at work, smoke only outdoors.

7. As soon as urge to smoke begins, start some alternative thing e.g., strike a conversation with somebody, start playing some music or busy your hand and mouth by some toothpicks.

8. Stop ending those associations of time and place which stimulate in you urge for smoking. Divert yourself from these to some other things or works or places. Stop visiting those places where smoking remains rampant.

9. Learn to relax. Join Yoga and meditation classes. These spiritual and health promoting practices will automatically develop in you the distaste for smoking over a period of time.

10. Go on collecting the money in a box which you will normally spend on cigarettes and count it on daily or weekly basis. This financial incentive will give you a further boost in stopping smoking.

Some interesting data/statistics on hazards of smoking

1. One in three cancer deaths is due to smoking.

2. One in five deaths from heart diseases is due to smoking.

3. Nine out of 10 deaths from bronchitis and emphysema (caused by lung damage) are a result of smoking.

4. The average smoker loses eight years of his life to cigarettes and has half the chance of reaching the age of 70 than someone who has never smoked.

5. Smokers have a 70% overall higher death rate as compared to non-smokers.

6. Possibility of coronary heart diseases is almost double in smokers as compared to non-smokers.

7. Sudden death may occur 4 times as commonly in young smokers as compared to their non-smoking counterparts. Among the males in age group of 40-54, the probability of premature death is 3 times more among smokers.

✿✿✿

Alcohol

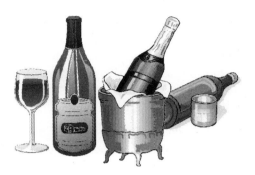

General characteristics

It is a colourless, volatile liquid known to the chemist as ethanol or ethyl Alcohol.

A number of alcoholic beverages in common use are derived from plants. Barley, grapes, rice and maize are some of the plants which yield alcoholic beverage. Following alcoholic beverages are commonly used—

1. **Beer:** It is formed from starch. Starch is changed into sugar which is fermented into alcohol by two distinct processes-malting and brewing. Barley is most commonly used. Alcohol content in beer is 3 to 8%.

2. **Wine:** It is produced by conversion of the sugar present in fruits of different varieties into alcohol and CO_2 through fermentation. Grapes are mainly used for making wine. Alcohol content in wine is 10 to 20%.

3. **Whisky:** Whisky is distilled from a fermented mash of malted or unmalted cereals or potatoes. Whisky contains 50% alcohol.

4. **Brandy:** It is distilled from white wine and has alcohol content of 56 to 60%.

43

5. **Rum:** It is distilled from juice and molasses of sugarcane and has alcohol content of 40%.

6. **Gin:** It is distilled from fermented mash of barley and rye meal. Alcohol content is 40%.

It can be seen from above that alcoholic beverages fall naturally into two classes—

a. **Fermented beverages:** in which alcohol is formed by the fermentation of sugar present either naturally in the source or produced by the transformation of starch as wine, e.g. Beer, Wine.

b. **Distilled beverages:** are obtained by the distillation of some alcoholic liquor, e.g. Whisky, Brandy, Rum, Gin.

Alcohol's direct action in the body seems to be limited strictly to one organ—the brain which controls the body's other activities. On this organ it acts as a depressant, not as the stimulant as it is commonly believed to be. Its depressant action, depending on the dose can cause mild or serious mental disorganisation, loss of muscular control (evident in slurred speech and staggering gait), sleep, coma and even death.

Journey of alcohol in the body

Alcohol, like most drugs, is carried to its target in the body by the blood. The route followed by alcohol is, of course, indirect. It is swallowed and reaches the blood stream by way of the gastro-intestinal tract, its first stop being the stomach. There, part of it passes into the blood vessels of the stomach wall. How much is absorbed in this way, and how fast, depends mainly on how dilute the alcohol is. A glass of beer (4 percent or more alcohol) or a dilute scotch (10 to 20 percent alcohol) are absorbed much more slowly than a straight shot of whisky (43 percent alcohol) and therefore produce far less of an immediate effect.

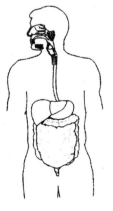

The greater part of the alcohol is not absorbed in the stomach at all but must wait until it passes into the small intestine. There its absorption is rapid, constant and complete. Thus, a major factor in how rapidly ingestion is followed by intoxication is how rapidly the alcohol passes from the stomach to the intestine. However food slows this passage, particularly proteins and fats, which being less easily digested remain in the stomach longest together with any alcohol mixed with them.

Effects of alcohol on consciousness at different concentrations

1. At a concentration in the blood of around .05%, (5 parts of alcohol to 1000 parts of blood), the effects of alcohol become noticeable, at least in the drinker's behaviour.

2. At 0.10%, the telltale signs of being "under the influence" include loud or slightly blurred speech and uncertain equilibrium and the drinker, in most countries, is legally presumed to be intoxicated, meaning that his ability to drive a car safely is considered to be significantly impaired.

3. At 0.20%, drinker will be staggering.

4. At 0.30%, drinker may be unable to stand.

5. At 0.40%, drinker will probably be unconscious and will therefore hardly be in a position to raise the level further.

6. An alcohol blood level of 0.50% to 0.60% is almost invariably fatal.

The above description is, of course, average. People vary in their response. The results of a given dose of alcohol also depend on the route it takes to the bloodstream, the speed at which it travels, the other substances it meets along the way and even the size of the body through which it is moving.

Sequence of effect of alcohol on brain centres

As has been mentioned earlier, alcohol seems to exert no direct effect on any organ except the brain even at high concentrations. It starts affecting different brain centres successively as follows.

1. **Effect on R.A.S.:** At smaller concentration, alcohol depresses the reticular activating system (RAS)—the part of the brain that alerts the cerebral cortex—the thinking and learning portion of the brain. Freed from control the cortex begins to function in a less organised manner. Activities requiring alertness, such as driving or concentration such as mathematical calculations are carried out less effectively. At the same time, ideas and images may flow more freely and less coherently.

2. **Blood circulation:** Alcohol affects the centre of the brain that controls the blood vessels. In the circulatory system, alcohol causes the capillaries that are situated just under the skin to dilate so that they carry more blood. The skin flushed with warm blood feels warmer. So does the drinker —but this, like many effects of alcohol, is an illusion. In fact, body temperature doesn't rise but falls, because much internal heat is carried by blood to the skin and dissipated there. Alcohol has never kept anyone warm in cold weather for a longer time. Indeed, in really cold weather it can lead to dangerous chilling. In hot climates, by contrast, the loss of body heat can be a boon.

   As a result of habitual heavy drinking, the dilation of the tiny capillaries can become permanent, producing the traditional flushed face and cherry nose.

3. **Kidneys:** Alcohol depresses a centre in the brain that normally slows the kidney's excretion of water. Hence alcohol speeds up excretion of water in the form of urine.

4. **Brain cortex:** At slightly higher concentration, alcohol extends its domain in the brain to the cortex itself whereby the finer grades of discrimination, memory, concentration and insight are dulled and then lost. Inhibitions are released with the result that the individual is likely to do and say things we would not do and say under normal

46

circumstances. For example he easily indulges in sex acts without shyness but his performance declines because of the dulling of sex centre in brain. Mood swings are uncontrolled and emotional outbursts frequent. Behaviour becomes impulsive because of impairment of faculty of judgement (Intellect).

5. **Cerebellum:** Still higher concentrations of alcohol depress more resistant parts of the brain. When the drug reaches the cerebellum which controls muscular coordination, the drinker's speech becomes garbled and his posture uncertain.

6. **Consciousness:** The next victims are the brain centres that control consciousness—at which point the drinker blacks out.

    Note: the deepest and most primitive portions of the brain, which keep the heart and lungs operating, are fortunately almost unaffected by any reasonable concentration of alcohol. Only the most determined and suicidal drinkers have managed to ingest enough of the drug to cause death from heart or respiratory failure.

Elimination of alcohol from the body

1. While alcohol is fogging the brain into intoxication, it is simultaneously being removed from the body.

2. A small portion of alcohol leaves the body unchanged through the lungs, skin and kidneys in the form of exhaled air, sweat and urine but all the rest is oxidised. Alcohol is combined with oxygen in the body and is ultimately transformed into carbondioxide and water. Since this change which is called oxidation is always accompanied by the production of energy, alcohol is a food as well as a drug. In fact we now know that a brandy or a glass of dry red table wine has about the same caloric value as a baked potato.

3. The organ that begins this job (oxidation) on alcohol is the liver. The first step in the transformation of alcohol in the liver is the drug's conversion into the compound acetaldehyde. This is even more toxic than alcohol. But luckily acetaldehyde is itself transformed almost immediately into a harmless compound, acetic acid (the

same substance that makes vinegar sour). At this point the liver's job ends, for acetic acid can be utilised by almost any cell of the body. But the liver remains the bottleneck, since it is only there that the crucial first steps can take place.

4. The body can't, under any circumstances, eliminate more alcohol than the liver can handle—about a quarter of an ounce an hour. If a person limited his alcohol intake to this amount—about half a shot of whisky or half a pint of beer per hour, he could drink indefinitely without getting drunk if he enjoyed that kind of activity. But an intake even slightly exceeding the liver's capacity will, sooner or later, build up intoxication.

When straight whisky is swallowed on an empty stomach, nearly all the alcohol is absorbed in a matter or minutes, almost before the body has time to begin eliminating and hence will cause more intoxication. The same amount of alcohol diluted in beer might be consumed and absorbed over an hour or more during which time a sizeable proportion of it would be eliminated, and hence will cause less intoxication.

5. The only effective remedy for intoxication is time. The liver's sluggish chemistry can't be substantially accelerated by any traditional treatment. But some symptoms of intoxication, such as sleepiness, can be alleviated by counteracting alcohol's depressant effects with a stimulant, thus fighting one poison with another. Most common of the stimulants is caffeine, in the form of strong coffee. The amphetamines (pep pills) are also used.

After effects of alcohol drinking

Once alcohol has disappeared from the body, it also has some aftereffects as listed below—

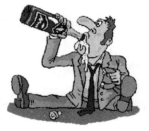

1. **Fatigue:** The most common symptom - fatigue has precisely the same cause as any other kind of

48

fatigue—overactivity. Alcohol, blocks off the mind's awareness of fatigue, so that the drinker is likely to cross the point at which he would otherwise succumb to exhaustion and sleep. On sobering up, he feels tired because he is tired.

2. **Headache:** The pounding hangover headache is partly the result of fatigue but also of changes in brain fluids brought about by alcohol.

3. **Nausea:** The nausea that frequently accompanies a hangover is apparently due partly to alcohol but also to its 'congeners'—chemicals of various sorts that become incorporated into alcoholic beverage during their manufacture. Liquors high in congeners, such as bourbon whisky are widely considered to have a greater hangover potential than congener in poor gin and vodka.

4. **Thirst:** The most universal hangover symptom of alcohol all over the world is the parched tongue and raging thirst that the French eloquently call "wooden month". Alcohol not only speeds up excretion of water, which of course induces thirst but also temporarily shifts some of the water remaining in the body from the interior of the cells to so the called extra cellular fluids. The partial dehydration of the cells affects the 'thirst centres' in brain, causing the hangover sufferer to feel more thirst than is warranted by his body's need for water.

Permanent harmful effects of alcohol on body

Unlike many drugs, alcohol doesn't seem to produce cumulative changes in the body, so long as it is consumed in moderate amounts. Despite the ominous preachments of prohibitionists, there is no proof that a life time of moderate indulgence interferes with normal health. But what happens is that people become addicted and continue to increase their intake because of the tolerance developed for the earlier doses. Such large amount of intake causes bodily damage as follows:

1. The most common form of cirrhosis, a disease that destroys cells of the liver, usually occurs in persistently heavy drinkers.

2. There is an extra strain on kidneys because kidneys have to excrete more water. Hence in later stage, kidneys may get damaged due to over exertion.

3. It produces gastritis or inflammation of the stomach. Strong alcohol (40%) irritates the gastric mucous membrane and increases the secretion of mucous. But it retards the secretion of gastric juice and gastric motility.

4. An alcoholic may develop severe symptoms of peripheral neuritis in which the nerves become weakened and deteriorated.

5. It produces a condition called 'wet brain' in which there is a marked swelling and congestion in the tissues covering the brain so that normal powers of coordination can no longer operate. It is said that everytime a person drinks, he loses some of his brain cells for ever.

6. It destroys various vitamins specially B & C.

7. Alcohol is a source of empty calories (without vitamins, minerals and proteins) and can be turned into fat, adding weight to the body. It increases the level of blood triglycerides and therefore indirectly affects the heart and increases blood pressure. However, there is a good news that moderate alcohol consumption increases HDL cholesterol (good cholesterol).

9. Decreased bone mass and condition of osteoporosis have been commonly observed in chronic alcoholics. This is because alcohol prevents the body from properly absorbing calcium and other important minerals.

10. Even in moderate dose, alcohol can lead to serious and occasionally lethal effects when it is taken in combination with certain other drugs. These include some sedatives such as barbiturates and many tranquilisers. Alcohol is a depressant and has an additive effect when combined with these. If an evening of heavy drinking is followed by the gulping of a

large number of barbiturate sleeping pills, the two drugs together may produce a fatal dose.

Smoking and alcohol

Many people who take alcohol also smoke. The combination has synergesic effect and creates manifold harm than their individual influence. The persons who drink more than 60 cc of alcohol a day along with smoking stand the risk of High B.P., stroke and heart attack.

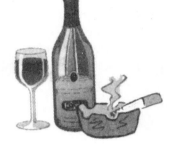

Liver identifies alcohol as a foreign substance and metabolises 95% of it into other chemicals. Liver can clear 15 cc of pure alcohol per hour. Alcoholic liver spends its precious hours in such work which remarkably reduces its capacity of doing other important metabolic functions. For example, the clearing of fat from blood is impaired. Hence lipids clog the blood stream. Simultaneously, chemicals from cigarette increase the coagulation of blood. This mechanism increases the chances of thrombus formation in coronary blood vessels. Tobacco contains 400 different chemicals which remain many more hours in blood stream in smokers who also take alcohol.

Withdrawal symptoms

Symptoms of alcohol withdrawal are closely comparable to the withdrawal syndrome expected with sedatives and hypnotics but the withdrawal symptoms are more common and severe in patients having poor health.

The symptoms may increase in severity for 3 to 4 days. The symptoms are those of hyperexcitability and may progress to a toxic psychosis characterised by marked alterations in perception and with auditory, visual and tactile hallucination.

Specific signs and symptoms include tremors, restlessness, agitation, insomnia, irritability, sweating, nausea, exaggerated reflexes and tachycardia. In severe cases delusions and hallucinations may occur.

Recommendations for alcoholics

1. An alcoholic should take plenty of fresh fruits and fruit juices in his diet.

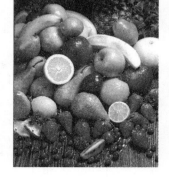

2. He should avoid strong condiments such as pepper, mustard and chilies.

3. He shouldn't smoke for this may only increase his desire for alcohol.

4. He should take multivitamin tablets particularly those containing the B-complex vitamins and ascorbic acid or vitamin C.

5. Alcohol for habitual consumers should be limited to 1 peg and not immediately stopped as it may lead to severe withdrawal symptoms as mentioned earlier.

✧✧✧

Refined Cereals

(White Flour, Polished Rice etc.)

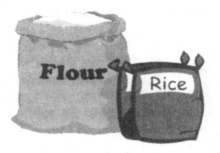

Refined cereals are mostly devoid of minerals, vitamins and fibres because these get lost when the outer husks of these cereals get removed in the refining process.

White flour (also called 'refined flour' or 'Maida') and polished rice are the two most widely used refined cereals in our day to day food. In the white flour, the outer husk of wheat called 'Wheat bran' is removed, while in polished rice the outer brown husk is removed during refining which are the major source of vitamins, minerals and fibres. Common white flour preparations which we use in our day to day life are white bread, naan, roomali roti, pizza, biscuits, cakes, noodles etc. Common polished rice preparations in our day to day life are pullao, biryani, plain and fried rice, dosa, etc.

Cereals contain mostly carbohydrates and after digestion and assimilation get converted into glucose just as any sugary food does. So by common sense we can say that refined cereals will also subject the body to most of the same harms which white sugar does, which is also devoid of any minerals, vitamins and fibres. However we will also separately list the predominant harms caused by refined cereals for greater understanding of the readers.

1. **Thiamine (Vit. B1) deficiency:** Vitamin B (specially Vit. B_1 known as thiamine) is necessary for digestion and assimilation by the body of all carbohydrate foods-the sugars and starches. None of the B–vitamins are present in refined cereals. Hence for assimilation and use of refined cereals by the body, the B–vitamins are stolen from nerves, muscles, liver, kidneys, stomach, heart, skin, eyes, blood etc. This leaves these organs of the body deficient in B–vitamins. Unless a large amount of food very rich in B–vitamins is taken, this deficiency will become worse and worse. As more of these refined foods is taken, more B–vitamins are stolen. We thus suffer from nervous irritability, digestive disorders, tiredness, poor eyesight, anaemia, heart trouble, muscular diseases, skin diseases etc. It may safely be said that many of such troubles would disappear if use of refined cereals like white flour, polished rice etc., is forbidden.

   If you eat carbohydrates in natural form, you don't experience 'thiamine' (Vit. B_1) deficiency because thiamine to digest the sugar or starch is present in the food. Thiamine is required for growth, good appetite and smooth functioning of digestive tract. A definite relation of thiamine deficiency to cardiac (heart) function has also been long recognised.

2. **Fatigue and depletion of energy:** Thinking that carbohydrates provide energy, people eat more and more refined cereals in the belief that they are going to get more and more energy. But this is actually not true because the thiamine deficiency in them (and if other sources of Vit. B_1 are also lacking in the body) won't allow the completion of carbohydrate metabolism and energy fails to be released properly and a by product called pyruvic acid accumulates in tissue cells and the result may be rather fatigue and less energy.

3. **Weakening of bones:** Carbohydrates for their metabolism require calcium. Since it is absent in refined cereals, this calcium is taken out of bones which will lead to weakening of bones leading sometimes to 'osteoporosis'.

4. **Lack of fibre:** These foods have no fibre. Hence they cause constipation.

5. **Increase in blood sugar:** Refined cereals lead to increase in blood sugar more rapidly than cereals with fibres. This is because fibre delays the absorption and assimilation.

Some situation where refined cereals can be consumed in moderation

1. Various combinations & supplementation is possible by use of refined cereals which can be occasionally taken e.g., Vegetable Sandwiches, Pizza with cheese, Vegetable & Paneer toppings, Vegetable Noodles with peas and omelette.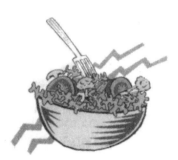

2. Idli made from semolina or sela rice is good. During fermentation, vitamin & mineral content is increased specially vitamin 'B'. Also sprouts and vegetables can be added to increase its nutrients.

3. Refined cereals are beneficial for those who require proteins restriction in their diets specially during kidney diseases.

4. Fiber rich biscuits, Atta biscuits, 'Rusk' etc. can be taken.

✿✿✿

Fatty Foods
and Cholesterol

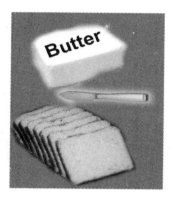

What is fat

Dietary fats and oils are combination of glycerol with fatty acids. One molecule of fat consists of three molecules of a fatty acid and one molecule of glycerol. That's why it is called triglycerides also. The storage fats of both plants (nuts and oilseeds) and animals are triglycerides. The fats are actually made up of the same three elements namely carbon, hydrogen and oxygen, of which the carbohydrates are made. The difference lies in the fact that fats contain less proportion of oxygen as compared to carbohydrates. Fats present in our foods can't be absorbed by our body as such. During the process of digestion, fat is broken down into fatty acid and glycerol.

Fats are members of a heterogeneous group of organic compounds known as lipids. The term lipid also includes, in addition to fat (or triglycerides), the cholesterol, cholesteryl esters and phospholipids. The common properties of all lipids are that (i) they all are esters of fatty acids (ii) they are insoluble in water (iii) they are soluble in nonpolar solvents such as ether, chloroform and benzene. Lipids are transported in blood as lipoproteins (Lipid-protein mix).

Requirement of fat in the body

1. Fat serves in the body as an efficient source of energy and for this purpose it is deposited in various fat depots (called adipose tissues) within the body and under the skin. In fact fats provide twice as much energy as that provided by the same amount of carbohydrates.

2. It serves as a thermal insulator in the subcutaneous tissues and around certain organs and also as electrical insulator.

3. Fats provide fat soluble vitamins (A, D, E, K) and are necessary for their absorption.

4. Fats give taste and flavour to the diet.

5. Combination of fat and protein (lipoproteins) are important cellular constituents, occurring both in the cell membrane and in the mitochondria within the cytoplasm and serving also as the means of transporting lipids in the blood.

6. Fats supply essential fatty acids to our body. Our body requires a large number of fatty acids for its functioning. However, most of these fatty acids needed by our body can be prepared from carbohydrates present in our body. But some of the fatty acids can't be synthesised by our body cells and must be supplied through the diet. These are called Essential Fatty Acids (EFA). These are two in number.

    a. **Linoleic acid:** Fatty acid containing 18 carbon atoms (chain length) and two double bonds. The first double bond is on the sixth carbon atom from the methyl (CH_3) end and therefore it is called n-6 fatty acid (or Omega 6 fatty acid).

    $$CH_3-(CH_2)_4-CH=CH-CH_2-CH=CH-(CH_2)_7-COOH$$

    b. **Alpha-linolenic acid:** Acid 18 carbon fatty acid with 3 double bonds. First double bond is on the third carbon atom from the methyl end and therefore it is called n-3 fatty acid (or Omega 3 fatty acid).

Essential Fatty acids are unsaturated fatty acids and are present in almost all plant foods and vegetable oils (except coconut oil).

Types of fats

Most natural fats are mixtures of saturated and unsaturated fats.

1. Saturated fats

Saturated fats contain saturated fatty acids (SFA). These fatty acids contain only single bonds in their carbon atoms and therefore have maximum number of hydrogen atoms that each carbon atom can carry. That's why they are called saturated fatty acids. All animal fats (with the exception of fish) are predominantly saturated fats, e.g. butter, ghee, cheese, milk, egg, meat. Saturated fats are in solid state at the room temperature as they have higher melting point.

Harmful effects of saturated fat: (i) Saturated fats increase blood cholesterol because of three reasons:

  a. First, they themselves contain cholesterol.

  b. Secondly, they stimulate the liver to produce more cholesterol.

  c. Thirdly, they inhibit the uptake of LDL cholesterol by cells i.e. cells can't take in cholesterol easily that is circulating in the blood.

(ii) Excess consumption will lead to increased level of triglycerides in blood and increased triglycerides storage in adipose tissue. This will lead to increase in body weight and problems connected with obesity. Excess blood triglycerides increase CHD risk also.

Benefits of saturated fats: (i) Foods cooked in saturated fats have a long shelf life because saturated fats are more stable and more resistant to oxidation.

(ii) They have a good smell and taste.

(iii) They provide fat soluble vitamins. Vit. E present in them functions as an antioxidant and delays the development of rancidity.

(iv) Saturated fats provide cholesterol. Some minimum amount of cholesterol is required by the body for its needs. Only excess is harmful.

2. Unsaturated fats

Fats containing unsaturated fatty acids are termed as unsaturated fats. Fatty acids containing one or more double bonds in their carbon atoms are called unsaturated fatty acids. Unsaturated fats tend to remain liquid at room temperature as they have comparatively low melting point. All vegetable oils (with the exception of palm and coconut oil) are predominantly unsaturated fats. In these fatty acids there is a shortage of hydrogen atoms. The carbon atoms then become linked by double bonds. That's why they are called unsaturated fatty acids. Due to the presence of double bonds, unsaturated fats are more reactive than saturated fats. Unsaturated fats are of two kinds—

    a. **Monounsatured fat:** Fatty acids having only one double bond in their carbon atoms are called Monounsaturated fatty acids (MUFA). For example Groundnut oil, mustard oil, olive oil and nuts (Almonds, cashewnuts, walnuts) contain MUFA. *Oleic acid* is the major fatty acid found in such fats.

    b. **Polyunsaturated fat:** contains fatty acids which have more than one double bonds in their carbon atoms, for example, sunflower oil, corn oil, safflower oil, cotton seed oil, soybeans oil etc., Linoleic and Alpha-Linolenic acids are the major fatty acids found in such fats.

Benefits of unsaturated fats: (i) Unlike SFA, both PUFA and MUFA reduce LDL (harmful) cholesterol.

(ii) In polyunsaturated fatty acids, omega 3 PUFA (n-3 PUFA) carries a special significance as it decreases blood triglycerides level and prevents clot formation by decreasing fibrinogen level and by inhibiting the activity of platelets. As mentioned earlier, Alpha linolenic acid in polyunsaturated fats get converted in the body to long chain n-3 PUFA. Plant foods such as wheat, black gram, rajmah, lobia, soyabean, pulses in general, spices such as mustard (rai), fenugreek seeds (methi) and green leafy vegetables are good sources of alpha-linolenic acid. In oils, mustard and soyabean oils are two common vegetable oils which contain alpha-linolenic acid. Similarly fish and fish oil are very rich source of Omega 3 polyunsaturated fatty acids (n-3 PUFA).

Harmful effects of unsaturated fats:

(i) Excess amount of PUFA may reduce HDL (good) cholesterol.

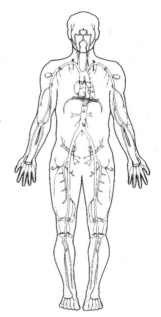

(ii) Though unsaturated fats reduce LDL (harmful) cholesterol but their excess consumption may increase blood triglycerides level as well as lead to weight gain in the body by deposit of these fats in adipose tissues.

(iii) Unsaturated fats are easily oxidised. Hence foods cooked in these fats tend to get rancid soon and have low shelf life.

It is now observed that triglycerides in blood above a particular limit also tend to deposit in arteries and tend to narrow and harden them. The increased body weight due to increased consumption of unsaturated fats may lead to problems of heart disease, diabetes and hypertension and also other diseases like gallstones, osteoarthritis and cancer.

3. Hydrogenated fats

The process by which unsaturated fats are converted into saturated fats by the addition of hydrogen at double bonds is called hydrogenation. At the same time it results in formation of trans fatty acid. Vanaspati ghee and margarine are two such fats.

Benefits of hydrogenated fats: Hydrogenation improves the appearance, shelf life and palatability of oils since they are not so easily oxidised as unsaturated fats. Hydrogenated fats are used in making commercially processed foods like biscuits and cakes.

Harmful effects of hydrogenated fat: Trans fatty acids raise LDL cholesterol, decrease HDL cholesterol and increase the tendency of abnormal blood clotting. Thus even though hydrogentated fats are devoid of any direct cholesterol in it, they are more detrimental for health compared to saturated fats obtained directly from animal sources.

CHOLESTEROL

What is cholesterol

Cholestrol is a soft waxy substance like fat (but not fat) which is produced mainly in the liver. It comes under the category of 'lipids'. It is important in the structure of body cells, hormones, bile acid and vitamin D. Hence, some amount of cholesterol is good for the body. Even when we consume no cholesterol, liver manufactures cholesterol in sufficient quantity for normal body functions.

Harmful effects of cholesterol

It is only the excess cholesterol generated in the body due to ill-planned diet which deposits in the lining of blood vessels and make them narrow and hardened, resulting in high blood pressure and other heart diseases. The process of narrowing and hardening of arteries due to deposition of cholesterol is called in medical parlance as 'Atherosclerosis'. Atherosclerosis also renders the blood vessels inelastic and brittle which makes artery easily susceptible to rupture. If a brittle brain artery ruptures, brain haemorrhage follows. This is termed as stroke. Stroke may lead to paralysis or instant death.

At the time of birth, arteries are smooth, open and elastic conduits for blood circulation. They expand and contract as blood flows through them. With ageing and wrong life-style and eating habits they lose their flexibility and become brittle by deposition of cholesterol. Calcium deposition may harden the arteries further. By narrowing of the arteries, blood flow is compromised to various organs. When the lumen of artery becomes narrow due to atherosclerosis, the chances of a blood clot or 'thrombus' being formed there becomes quite high. If such blood clot blocks a coronary artery, it may result in a heart attack or severe angina. If a blood clot is formed in brain artery, it may lead to brain haemorrhage or stroke. Blood clot is formed by platelets, red blood cells and other cells sticking together.

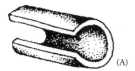

(A)

Healthy artery: In early Childhood, the artery walls are free of any damage. The risk of heart attack is also low.

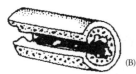

(B)

Atherosclerosis: In later years Arteries become clogged with plaque due to factors such as excessive cholesterol.

Deposits of Cholesterol

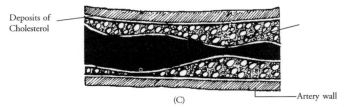

Artery wall

(C)

Longitudinal cross-section of an artery showing variation of cholesterol deposition along the artery wall.

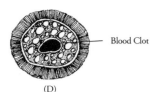

Blood Clot

(D)

Blood clot formation in the constricted area of artery.

Since the walls of the arteries also become roughened in atherosclerosis, the blood cells easily adhere there and form blood clots.

How cholesterol is carried in blood

Let us understand how cholesterol travels in the blood stream. Fats and cholesterol are carried in the blood in the form of Lipoproteins. There are three kinds of Lipoproteins -

1. VLDL (Very Low Density Lipoprotein)

2. LDL (Low Density Lipoprotein)

3. HDL (High Density Lipoprotein)

VLDL is not much important as far as cholesterol is concerned. Cholesterol attached to LDL is called LDL cholesterol (LDL-C). Cholesterol attached to HDL is called HDL cholesterol (HDL-C).

Through LDL, cholesterol is carried via blood stream to the cells and tissues. Through HDL, excess cholesterol is carried back to liver via blood stream.

If ratio of LDL-C and HDL-C is not within limits, then excess cholesterol which is not used by cells remains in the blood stream and sticks to artery's walls leading to thickening and hardening of arteries.

HDL cholesterol is considered to be good cholesterol because it is protective and helpful. It rather reduces harmful LDL cholesterol from the blood and tissues and delivers it back to the liver where it is processed for excretion.

It is the LDL cholesterol which is the main culprit promoting deposits in the arteries and gradually blocking the passage for blood. Hence it is desirable to have higher HDL and lower LDL cholesterol in blood.

Triglycerides

Previously it was thought that unlike cholesterol, triglycerides (fats) don't deposit in the lining of arteries. But new researches show that triglycerides also start depositing in the arteries, if present excessively. Triglycerides are fats devoid of any cholesterol. The stored fats of both plants (nuts and oil seeds) and animals (depot fats) are triglycerides. That's why it is desirable to have regulated intake of unsaturated fats also (which is devoid of any cholesterol) since they will increase blood triglyceride level. Triglycerides and cholesterol together are called blood lipids.

Ways to reduce triglyceride level

1. Reduce total fat intake.
2. Reduce sugar, sweets and soft drinks (as excess sugar readily gets converted to triglycerides in the body).
3. Reduce alcohol intake. Alcohol increases triglyceride level of blood.
4. Do regular exercises. They help to reduce blood triglyceride level.
5. Increase intake of Omega 3 PUFA rich foods (or Alpha linolenic acid) as they reduce blood triglyceride level. For the benefit of readers, sources of such foods are given below:

    i.   **Cereals and millets:** wheat, bajra
    ii. **Pulses & legumes:** Blackgram, Urad, Lobia, Rajmah, Soyabean, Bengalgram (kalachana)
    iii. **Vegetables:** Green leafy vegetables
    iv. **Spices:** Fenugreek (Methi), Mustard (rai)
    v.   **Oils:** Mustard, Soyabean
    vi. **Animal food:** fish

6. Do occasional fasting. Fasting reduces blood triglyceride level.

Ways to increase HDL (good) cholesterol

1. Do regular exercises. Exercise increases HDL cholesterol.
2. Reduce total fat intake. There is a reciprocal relationship between blood levels of triglycerides level and HDL cholesterol. Hence people with high blood triglycerides tend to have low HDL.

3. Reduce intake of transfatty acids (Vanaspati ghee, Margarine). They reduce HDL cholesterol.

4. Reduce excessive intake of PUFA-rich oils. HDL levels may decrease if PUF accounts for more than 10% of energy intake.

5. Certain foods have been found to improve HDL cholesterol e.g., onion, soyabean, garlic, soluble fibre (e.g. 'pectin' in apple), banana, Isabgol powder etc.

Ways to reduce LDL (harmful) cholesterol

1. Reduce saturated fat intake and increase unsaturated fat (MUFA & PUFA) intake.

2. Reduce intake of dietary cholesterol. Foods having high cholesterol should be avoided. (see tables at the end of this chapter).

3. Reduce intake of tea, coffee, soft drinks, chocolate etc. The caffeine in these products stimulates excess cholesterol production in the body.

4. Reduce intake of tobacco (smoking, pan chewing etc.)

5. Reduce mental stress. Stress has been found to increase LDL cholesterol.

6. Avoid sedentary life and do regular exercises.

7. Take measures to cure high blood pressure and diabetes if you have any of these diseases since these diseases tend to increase cholesterol in blood.

8. Increase intake of foods containing soluble fibres e.g. apple, banana, carrot, potato, oat bran, pulses, Isabgol etc. Soluble fibre binds with dietary cholesterol and is excreted out of the body alongwith undigested food.

9. Certain foods have been found to reduce LDL cholesterol, for example, onion, garlic, soybeans, Amla etc. It is observed that daily intake of 3-4 cloves of fresh garlic and Amla (in any form—Juice or raw or pickle) have substantial cholesterol lowering effect.

Some recommendations for using vegetable oils

1. Choose a variety of vegetable oils instead of a single oil since most of the vegetable oils don't have an ideal mix of PUFA, MUFA and Omega 3 PUFA in them. (Note-oils with only high PUFA are not desirable since they reduce HDL cholesterol)

2. Mix two or more oils of different composition. A good choice is equal mixture of PUFA rich sunflower, safflower or corn oil and MUFA rich groundnut oil. Vegetarians may supplement this mixture with occasional use of mustard oil to ensure omega 3 PUFA intake. Mustard oil alone is not a good choice since it contains erucic acid which is detrimental for health. Sesame oil is good since it contains nearly equal amount of PUFA and MUFA.

3. Vegetable oils undergo chemical changes on exposure to air, high temperature and humidity, hence, following precautions should be observed in their purchase and storage:

    i.   Purchase always a fresh batch of the oil by checking the date of manufacture.

    ii. Select a packing which is likely to be consumed within a month.

    iii. Prefer aluminium or coloured glass packing over plastic or tin.

    iv. Remove the oil from plastic or tin container at home and refill the oil in an airtight and waterproof steel, aluminium or an opaque glass bottle.

    v.   Don't leave the lid of the oil container open since it will tend to react with air.

    vi. Keep the oil in refrigerator during peak summer and rainy season.

Some important facts regarding fats and cholesterol summarised

1. Some amount of fat intake is necessary for the body. Zero fat diet is harmful for the body. It is the excess fat

and wrong combination and type of fats which are harmful for the body.

2. Saturated fats increase blood cholesterol and triglycerides.

3. Transfatty acids increase blood cholesterol, reduce HDL cholesterol and increase blood clotting tendency.

4. Vegetable oils and all plant foods don't have cholesterol (except palm and coconut).

5. Monounsaturated fats (MUFA) decrease blood cholesterol.

6. Polyunsaturated fats (PUFA) decrease blood cholesterol.

7. Omega 3 fatty acids present in some PUFA reduce triglycerides, prevent clot formation and reduce LDL cholesterol.

8. Excess of PUFA decreases HDL (good) cholesterol.

9. Fish and fish oils lower blood triglycerides, prevent clot formation and decrease LDL cholesterol.

10. Animal foods have saturated fats and have substantial cholesterol (except fish).

11. Carbohydrates particularly refined sugars have no cholesterol but they increase triglycerides.

12. Soluble fibres (found in cereals, pulses, vegetables, fruits) decrease cholesterol and triglycerides.

13. Daily intake of cholesterol for a normal person shouldn't exceed 300 mg/day and for persons with coronary heart diseases (CHD), it should not be more than 200 mg/day.

14. Excess of PUFA increases blood triglyceride level.

15. Alcohol increases blood triglyceride level. Its moderate amount increases HDL (good) cholesterol level also.

16. Some amount of cholesterol is needed by body for its functioning. Hence a limited intake of saturated fats is not harmful.

SOME USEFUL TABLES

Table 1

Blood Lipids Chart (mg/100 ml plasma)

Type of lipids	Desirable	Borderline High	High Risk
Total Cholesterol	<200	200-240	>240
LDL Cholesterol	<130	130-160	>160
HDL Cholesterol	>50	50-35	<35
Triglycerides	<150	150-500	>500

Table 2

Foods Containing Saturated and Unsaturated Fats

Food containing mainly saturated fats	Foods containing mainly unsaturated fats
a. Butter, ghee (clarified butter), vegetable ghee (vanaspati ghee or Dalda, coconut oil, palm oil)	a. Vegetable oils: Peanut oil, sesame oil, maize oil, soyabean oil, karadi oil, cottonseed oil, sunflower oil, and dishes prepared from these oils
b. Whole milk, cream, khoya, khoya-based preparations, sweets prepared in ghee and vegetable ghee, whole-milk preparations (shreekhand, basudi, ice cream, pedas, etc.), Cheese	b. Nuts: Almonds, Cashewnuts, Peanuts, Walnuts, Pistachio etc.
c. Chocolates, cakes, biscuits, wafers	c. Invisible fats from cereals, pulses, vegetables etc.
d. Egg, meat	

Table 3

Fat Contents of Commonly Used Vegetable Oil & Ghee (in%)

Oils & Ghee	Satur-ated Fat	Monoun-satura-ted Fat (Oleic Acid)	Poly-unsaturated Fat Lino-leic Acid	Alpha Linol-enic Acid	Predomi-nant Fatty Acids
Coconut	90	7	2	<0.5	Saturated
Palm Kernel	82	15	2	<0.5	Saturated
Ghee	65	32	2	<1.0	Saturated
Vanaspati	24	19	3	<0.5	Saturated
Red Palm Oil (raw)	50	40	9	<0.5	Saturated +Monoun-saturated
Palm oil	45	44	10	0.5	Saturated +Monoun-saturated
Olive	13	76	10	<0.5	Monoun-saturated
Groundnut	24	50	25	<0.5	Monoun-saturated
Rape /Mustard	8	70	12	1.0	Monoun-saturated
Sesame	15	42	42	1.0	Mono and Polyun-saturated
Rice bran	22	41	35	1.5	Mono and Polyun-saturated

contd...

Oils & Ghee	Saturated Fat	Monounsaturated Fat	Polyunsaturated Fat		Predominant Fatty Acids
		(Oleic Acid)	Linoleic Acid	Alpha Linolenic Acid	
Cotton seed	22	25	52	1.0	Polyun-saturated
Corn	12	32	55	1.0	Polyun-saturated
Sunflower	13	27	60	<0.5	Polyun-saturated
Safflower	13	17	70	<0.5	Polyun-saturated
Soyabean	15	27	53	5.0	Polyun-saturated

Table 4

Fat & Cholesterol Content of Various Foods
(per 100 gm of food)

Name of food	Fat (gm)	Cholesterol (mg)
Cereals & Pulses		
White flour	1.4	0
Rice	0.6	0
Daal	1.5	0
Oats	7.0	0
Vegetables & Fruits		
Green vegetables	0.3	0
Fruits	0.0	0

contd...

Name of food	Fat (gm)	Cholesterol (mg)
Fats & Oils		
Butter	80	240
Desi Ghee (clarified butter)	98	310
Vegetable oil	99	0
Margarine	99.8	0
Nuts		
Almonds	56	0
Walnuts	67	0
Cashewnuts	55.6	0
Peanuts	56	0
Pistachio nuts	54.5	0
Milk & Milk products		
Ice cream	10	41
Kulfi	15	30
Paneer (buffalo)	31.2	124
Milk (cow)	4	14
Milk (buffalo)	8	16
Milk (skimmed)	0.1	2
Milk (condensed)	10	40
Cream	13	40
Cheese (Cheddar)	25	100
Egg		
Egg (whole)	11	400
Egg yolk	30	1120
Meat		
Chicken without skin	4	60
Chicken with skin	18	100

contd...

Name of food	Fat (gm)	Cholesterol (mg)
Beef	16	70
Mutton	13	65
Pork	35	90
Organ meats		
Brain	6	2000
Heart	5	150
Kidney	2	370
Liver	9	300
Sea foods		
Prawn/shrimps	2	150
Fish (lean)	1.5	45
Fish (fatty)	6	45

Table 5

Cholesterol Counter in Convenient Measures

Item	Quantity	Cholesterol (mg)
Whole milk	1 glass	50
Ice Cream	1 cup	84
Whole egg (or egg yolk)	1 no.	210
Butter	1 tbsp	36
Skimmed milk	1 glass	7
Frozen yoghurt	1 cup	10
Egg white	1 no.	0
Cream	1 cup	180

1 tbsp (tablespoon) = 15 ml
1 cup (big) = 210 ml
1 glass = 300 ml   ✿✿✿

72

Fried Foods

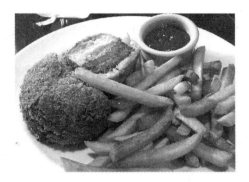

We are daily consuming fried foods in one form or the other, e.g. cutlets, tikkis, pakoras, samosas, poories, paranthas, french fries, chips, gulab jamuns, omelettes etc. Frying refers to cooking of food in plenty of hot oil so that item is largely immersed in the oil or floats over it. Fried foods cause lot of harmful effects in our body as mentioned below:

1. **High fat content:** Fried foods have high fat content and are energy dense. A regular consumption of fried foods may lead to fat intake far in excess of body demands. For example, a medium size poorie provides 2.2 gm fat and 70 Kcal of energy. A chapati made from the same amount of flour has only 51 Kcal and unless ghee is applied, the amount of fat in it is negligible. A vegetable cutlet provides as much as 100 Kcal and 3.3 gms of fat. It leads to undesirable weight gain.

2. **Chemical changes in oil and formation of harmful chemicals:** Frying leads to undesirable alteration in chemical composition of oils. Chemical changes are more when oils are exposed to intense heat during deep frying.

Heating edible oils beyond certain temperatures results in formation of several volatile as well as nonvolatile decomposition products. Volatile decomposition products (VDP) are inhaled by the cook during food preparation. After food preparation, VDP residues also persist in leftover oil. If such oil is reused, VDP find their way to the gut of the consumer. VDP irritate and damage the inner lining of the gut which may cause bowel upset manifesting as abdominal pain, nausea, vomiting or diarrhoea.

On frying, foods release their moisture in oil. Heat induced decomposition of oils is accelerated by this moisture. Moisture agitates hot oil, thereby hastening its chemical breakdown.

Prolonged heating results in formation of several other harmful chemicals in oil, one of which *is acrolein*, which besides irritating the gut lining, may also be a cancer causing compound. Prolonged or repeated heating of polyunsaturated fats also produce toxic substances such as polymerized products, peroxides, free radicals etc. Harmful effects of these are explained in a separate note on free radicals at the end of chapter.

It is also to be noted that Polyunsaturated fats are more easily oxidised compared to saturated fats. Saturated fats are resistant to oxidation even at frying temperatures. This is why foods cooked in saturated fats (e.g. ghee) have long shelf life.

3. **Formation of Trans-fatty acid:** At high temperature, natural form of fats may undergo change into trans-form. Trans-fatty acids increase blood cholesterol levels even more than desi ghee or other animal fats do. They also reduce HDL (good) cholesterol and increase the tendency of blood clotting, thus increasing the risk of coronary heart disease (CHD).

4. **Loss of Nutrients:** Frying exposes oil to much higher temperature. At these temperatures many nutrients, especially vitamins, are destroyed and dietary proteins are

adversely affected. Beyond 150°C, there is progressive decrease in vitamin A and E content of oil.

5. **Difficult to digest and delayed stomach emptying:** Fried foods with their high fat content lead to delayed stomach emptying. They are heavy and not so easily digested as foods which are boiled, baked or steamed. They are not suitable for persons suffering from indigestion.

Some recommendations

If you are using fried foods occasionally, taking the following precautions will reduce the damage caused by them.

1. Oil with high smoking point should be chosen for frying. Smoking point of an oil is the temperature at which it starts emitting a blue haze indicating formation of decomposition products. The minimum temperature necessary for frying is around 200°C. Therefore fats with smoking point more than 220°C are suitable for frying. Most vegetable cooking oils have adequately high smoking points. Pure ghee has an intermediate smoking point. Butter and coconut oil are not suitable for frying due to low smoking point.

2. Foods should be fried at optimum temperature, say nearly 200°C. When frying temperature is too low, food tends to absorb too much oil. Frying at very high temp. often leads to browning of the surface while the core may still be raw.

3. Use a non-stick 'pan', 'Tawa', 'Karahi' for frying. Fat content of fried foods can be somewhat controlled by using them.

4. Don't reheat the oil. Oils are often heated for long duration at high temperature and used repeatedly during frying operation. This is not desirable. Heating the oil lowers its smoking point. Frying foods with low smoking point oils also leaves the product raw from inside even though the surface has turned brown.

It is better to use the minimum possible quantity of the oil for frying to avoid wastage and it should be heated only when raw material is ready for cooking.

Ideally, oil should be discarded after one time use. However, if economy doesn't permit, used oil should be stored in a refrigerator till such time it is reused. It should be filtered before storage so as to remove the burnt food particles in it which otherwise will cause deterioration in oil quality. Oil shouldn't be stored for long before it is used again.

5. Drain excess of oil. It may be a good idea to put fried food on an oil absorbent paper (e.g. tissue paper) and press it between the folds to remove excess oil before eating.

Note on free radical

It was mentioned earlier that frying and prolonged heating leads to formation of free radicals. This word has now come into great prominence and it has a great bearing on our health, so I will like to explain it in more detail.

A free radical is an unstable oxygen molecule with an unpaired electron. In the absence of a pairing electron, free radical turns very reactive and has the potential of causing severe damage to the cell structure such as its membrane, its fat, its protein and the DNA and RNA. These free radicals can potentially induce cancer, heart disease, inflammation in the arthritic joint, brain degeneration and could damage the brain cells to the extent of senility. These free radicals accelerate the aging process. Ageing occurs when our cells are permanently damaged due to continuous attack from these free radicals. These free radicals also oxide several blood constituents including those harmful LDL. These oxidised lipids are more likely to be deposited in artery walls than unoxidised lipids. In technical language we say that free radicals subject the body to oxidative stress.

It is to be noted that frying or prolonged heating of oil is not the only process in which free radicals are generated but there are many other sources of free radicals also which are given below for the information of inquisitive readers—

1. Smoking
2. Air pollution
3. Car exhaust fumes
4. Exposure to sunlight (UV radiation)
5. Stress
6. Insecticides and pesticide chemicals in foods
7. Radiation from air travel
8. Radiation from computer screens
9. Microwave ovens
10. Electric blankets
11. Television sets
12. X-rays
13. High voltage wiring in overhead pylons
14. Fluorescent lighting

Free radicals are also being formed daily in our body through normal body processes of metabolism when oxygen is burnt as fuel in our cells.

Body has an inbuilt system to neutralise these free radicals as much as possible through its store of antioxidants which can give up one of their electrons but without becoming an unstable molecule themselves. As long as the body has a sufficiently high antioxidant status, it can keep the production and damaging effects of free radicals in check.

Since antioxidants can repair free radical damage, it makes sense to have a great deal of them around you. These are abundant in fruits and vegetables. The most powerful antioxidants are Vit. A, C & E. Others include Selenium, Chromium, Zinc and Calcium. Fruits/vegetables which are yellow, orange and green in colour are the principal dietary sources of antioxidants and other micronutrients. In fruits/vegetables, darker the colour the higher the vitamin and mineral content. Onion and garlic are also said to be good antioxidants. Antioxidants infuse into each cell and intercept/neutralise the free radical activity.

One must avoid sugar and fats in excess as they are easily oxidised by free radicals. Free radicals attack fats that are ingested in food thereby turning them rancid.

So, in short, by taking plenty of fruits and vegetables, having antioxidant vitamins A, C & E (e.g., carrots, lettuce, oranges etc.), by cutting down sugar and fats, by keeping away from various sources of free radicals as mentioned above and by exercising regularly, one can save himself considerably from free radical damage.

For the benefit of readers, we are mentioning below the various sources of Vit. A, C & E.

Vit. A: Milk, butter, ghee, carrot, mango, papaya, orange, green leafy vegetables, egg, fish, liver, orange, tomato, apricot.

Vit. C: Amla, lemon, orange, tomatoes, guava, cabbage, mosambi, potato, watermelon, pineapple, green leafy vegetables, grapefruit, mango, strawberry, cauliflower, Plum, Papaya, Green chillies.

Vit. E: Vegetable oils and seeds, green leafy vegetables, almonds, peanuts, walnuts, egg yolk, cereals (specially whole grain wheat flour, wheat germ), milk, butter, onion, garlic, avocados, plums, corn, spinach, banana, pumpkin, tomato, lettuce, sweet potato (sakargandi).

✿✿✿

Non-Vegetarian Foods

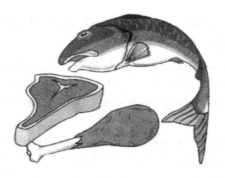

F ollowing harmful effects have been observed in the non-vegetarian foods—

1. Meat or animal foods have large amount of saturated fats and contain lot of cholesterol. This cholesterol brings about hardening and narrowing of arteries (atherosclerosis) leading to High B.P. and other heart diseases. Too much fat also leads to problems of weight gain and obesity.

2. Protein obtained from meat has high uric acid. It leads to problems of arthritis, gout etc. This can also lead to kidney failure because kidneys have to overwork to remove the uric acid.

3. Meat has low dietary fibre. This leads to colonic disorders, constipation etc.

4. Meat is considered a 'Tamsik' food. It creates inertia, heaviness and dullness in the body since its digestion takes more time and body has to expend more energy in the digestion of meat or non-veg foods.

5. If the animal is diseased or the meat is infected, eating such a meat may lead to food poisoning and disease in the body and sometimes even cancer of the colon.

6. Although from the point of view of composition and ratio of various amino acids, animal protein is considered better than vegetable protein but this deficiency can be made up by choosing a judicious combination of vegetable foods, e.g. soyabeans, nuts, milk and pulses can give us a high class protein.

7. Meats are highly acidic food and create problem of acidity in the body.

8. When an animal is killed, it cries with pain and is highly scared. This leads to release of many toxins and chemicals in its body which are ingested by us when we eat its meat.

   Spiritually it is said that the negative vibrations of the suffering animal permeate its body when it is killed and when we eat its flesh, the same vibrations affect our psyche and soul accordingly.

9. Since meat is always eaten of a dead animal, its prana or vitality is considerably lost. That is why meat eaters inspite of taking so much fat always feel exhausted and drained of energy and they have little stamina and endurance.

   It is to be noted that there is a fundamental difference between humans and carnivorous animals. The former have an alkaline stomach and the latter have highly acidic stomach where even the raw flesh will get dissolved on its way to digestion.

A few words about fish

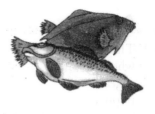

Among non-vegetarian foods, fish is considered to have some beneficial qualities because of which its limited consumption is not considered bad. For example:

1. Fish is a good source of Omega 3 fatty acids (n-3 PUFA) which make the blood less prone to abnormal clotting process because these fatty acids inhibit the activity of

platelets and decrease the fibrinogen level. In addition these fatty acids reduce the blood levels of cholesterol and triglycerides and increase good (HDL) cholesterol.

2. Its high potassium keeps the blood pressure in a reasonable range.

3. Most fish are high in potassium, phosphorus, magnesium, zinc and A, B & D vitamins. Fish is also rich in iron and it is in a form that is easier to absorb than iron from the plant sources.

4. Fish contains an amino acid 'tyrosin'. It helps make such chemicals in the body which energise the brain.

5. Cod liver oil is very effective in treating arthritis and rheumatism.

However like most other non-vegetarian foods, fish also increases acidity, uric acid and blood urea with consequential adverse effects. Consumption of certain vegetarian foods can give all the benefits accruing from the consumption of fish minus its acidity and blood urea. Hence, in conclusion we can say that if it is not possible to take totally vegetarian food, then eating fish in small quantities to the exclusion of other non-vegetarian foods like mutton, beef, pork, chicken, poultry is suggested. There are many varieties of fish, e.g. shell fish, oysters, clams, shrimps, shark, cod, salmon, sardines, trout, rahu, seer, purava and hilsa etc. from which to choose from Fishes can be of white and black type, lean and fatty type, fresh water and sea water type etc.

A few words about egg

There has always been a controversy whether egg is a non-vegetarian food or vegetarian food or an in-between category popularly known as 'eggetarian'. Whatever be the case, it has been proved that 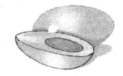 compared to other non-vegetarian food, egg really has an edge over them and many researchers even call it a near complete food. Let us ponder over salient features of an egg.

1. Egg consists of three portions—Egg white, egg yolk, egg shell (outer covering). Calcium content of egg is mostly in the outer covering or shell which is not consumed by human. However the chick embryo is able to obtain calcium from the egg shell. But the other minerals like sodium, potassium, magnesium, iron and zinc are present in the edible portion of egg as mentioned in the table ahead.

2. Egg protein is considered to be a very good quality protein. It has 6.2 gm protein, nearly half of which is present in egg yolk. It used as a standard against which the quality of other protein sources is assessed (see table ahead). Milk, milk products and meat proteins also have high biological value. The biological value of a protein is a measure of how efficiently the food protein can be converted into body tissues. And that depends on the closeness of its amino acid composition to the pattern in body tissues.

   It can be seen from the table ahead that some vegetarian foods like soyabean, peas, peanuts, etc. also provide good quality proteins and can serve as egg substitutes if one doesn't take egg.

3. Egg contains significant amounts of vitamins A,B,D & E (see table ahead). Egg is an excellent source of vitamin B_{12} which is vital for the nervous system.

4. Egg has high cholesterol content and it is easy to believe that consumption of egg will always increase blood cholesterol. However the research has shown that this relationship is not really so straight forward. It has been observed that increase in blood cholesterol level occurs more readily not by dietary cholesterol but by dietary saturated fats which promote excessive blood cholesterol manufacture by the liver.

   It is to be noted that eggs are low in fat. One egg contains about 5 gm. fat of which less than 2 gm. is saturated. Therefore the increase in blood cholesterol level with modest egg intake is much smaller compared to other flesh foods and dairy products which are rich sources of saturated fats in addition to dietary cholesterol. Therefore relatively high cholesterol content of egg is only of concern to people who already have raised blood cholesterol levels.

5. Egg doesn't contain vitamin C. Egg also doesn't provide complex carbohydrates and fibres. Hence for patients having diabetes, heart diseases and obesity, it is not much beneficial.

6. Sometimes egg becomes infectious. This is because its outer covering or shell contains microbes, dirt etc. Which can be removed only if washed properly. Egg vendors don't keep it washed because it will reduce the quality of egg. While buying, always reject any eggs that have cracked or blemished shells.

7. The quality of egg deteriorates with storing. While buying, it is not known whether the egg is stale or fresh until it is tested in laboratory. The quality of nutrients present in egg goes on reducing as the egg gets stale.

8. In some people, egg causes food allergy.

9. Eggs have protein name 'Evidin'. This protein inactivates a vitamin named 'Biotin' (a vitamin of B-complex group). This sometimes leads to pain in muscles, skin disorders etc.

10. There is a risk of 'salmonella' poisoning in egg, if not thoroughly cooked. However it is observed that only one egg in every 7000 harbours salmonella bacteria (which are passed on by the hen and are not due to unhygienic living conditions). But to avoid any eventuality, avoid eating raw eggs in any form. Egg must be cooked properly to destroy bacteria. To be absolutely certain, you must boil eggs for atleast 7 minutes. Both the yolk and the white should be firm. Omelettes should be cooked until dry.

11. *Lecithin* in egg yolks is rich in *choline*, which is involved in the transport of cholesterol in the bloodstream and in fat metabolism. It is also an essential component of cell

membranes and nervous tissue. Even though the body is able to make enough *choline* for its normal needs, additional amount provided by diet may be helpful in treating the accumulation of fat in the liver, as well as certain types of neurological damage.

How many eggs to be eaten

How many eggs is it safe to eat before the cholesterol contained in their yolks becomes a problem? The British Heart Foundation recommends eating no more than four eggs a week.

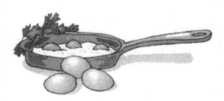

Composition of Hen's Egg

	Whole Egg	Egg White	Egg Yolk
Weight (gm)	50.0	33.4	16.6
Energy (Kcal)	75.0	17.0	59.0
Protein (gm.)	6.25	3.52	2.78
Carbohydrate (gm)	0.61	0.34	0.30
Fat (gm)	5.01	0.0	5.12
Cholesterol (mg)	213.0	0.0	213.0
Saturated Fats (gm)	1.55	0.0	1.59
Monounsaturated Fats (gm)	1.91	0.0	1.95
Polyunsaturated Fats (gm)	0.682	0.0	0.698
Sodium (mg)	63.0	55.0	7.0
Potassium (mg)	60.0	48.0	16.0
Magnesium (mg)	5.0	4.0	1.0
Iron (mg)	0.72	0.01	0.59

contd...

	Whole Egg	Egg White	Egg Yolk
Zinc (mg)	0.55	0.0	0.52
Vitamin A (mg)	95.2	0.0	97.0
Vitamin C (mg)	0.0	0.0	0.0
Thiamin (mg)	0.031	0.002	0.028
Riboflavin (mg)	0.254	0.151	0.106
Niacin (mg)	0.037	0.031	0.002
Vitamin B_6 (mg)	0.07	0.001	0.065
Folic Acid (Micro gm)	23.0	1.0	24.0
Vitamin B_{12} (Micro gm)	0.5	0.07	0.052
Calcium (mg)	25.0	2.0	23.0
Phosphorous (mg)	89.0	4.0	81.0
Selenium (mg)	0.022	0.005	0.007
Fibre (gm)	0.0	0.0	0.0
Vitamin E (mg)	0.7	0.0	0.7

Biological Value of Selected Food Proteins

Food	Biological value of Protein
Egg	100
Cow's Milk	93
Fish	76
Unpolished Rice	86
Groundnut	55
Whole Wheat	65
Corn	72
Soyabean	73
Peas	64

✿✿✿

Acidic Foods

Our blood is basically alkaline in nature. To maintain its alkalinity, we need 80% alkaline foods and 20% acid forming foods. Some of our foods leave alkaline residues in the body after undergoing the full cycle of digestive and metabolic processes, some others leave acidic residues. We may call such foods alkali-genic and acid-genic respectively.

Generally the acids produced by the metabolic activities (such as uric acid, lactic acid etc.) react with alkalis in the blood, lymph, bile etc., thus being neutralised. But if our diet is flooded with acid-genic foods, the body can't cope with all the resulting acids and the symptoms of fatigue, headache, anorexia, insomnia, nervous tension, hyperacidity, coryza etc. begin to appear.

There are other important side effects in the body due to increased acidity of the blood. The body uses sodium as a buffer to help bring an acidic pH back to normal for maintenance of homeostasis in body, whereby sodium becomes depleted. When sodium can no longer adequately buffer accumulated acid, the body uses calcium as a second buffer. This calcium is leached from bones and teeth if our diet doesn't contain enough of it. This results in weakening of bones and bones become porous and brittle. This problem in medical parlance is known as 'Osteoporosis'.

Chronic acidity is an unhealthy condition and causes faster degeneration and ageing in the body. All the toxic substances in the body are in the form of acids and in order to prevent or counteract the accumulation of acids in the body we must take foods which are mainly alkaline in nature.

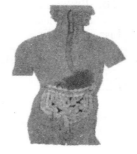

Hence it is important to know first as to which foods are acidgenic and which foods are alkaline in nature. Foods are classified as acid producing or alkali producing depending on their final end products in the body after metabolism. Calcium, magnesium, sodium, iron, copper, manganese and potassium present in food contribute to the alkaline effects while sulphur, phosphorus, chlorine, iodine, carbondioxide and carbonic, lactic and uric acids present in foods contribute to the acidic effect.

List of acidic foods

1. **All animal foods:** Meat, egg, fish, chicken etc.

2. **Dairy products:** Heated and pasteurised milk, cheese, curd and butter.

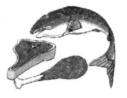

3. **Dried peas and beans**

4. **All cereals and pulses:** wheat, maize, rice etc., and pulses.

5. **All nuts and seeds (dried):** Peanut, walnut, cashewnut, sesame, sunflower, melon seeds.

6. **All processed foods:** white bread, biscuits, bakery products, white flour, polished rice, white sugar.

7. **Toxic foods:** Tea, Coffee, Alcohol, Tobacco, Soft drinks.

8. **All fats and oils.**

9. **All fried and spicy foods.**

10. **All sugary foods & sweets (Containing white sugar).**

List of alkaline foods

1. All fruits (fresh or dried) including citrus fruits.

2. All green, leafy and root vegetables (except peas & beans).

3. Sprouts of beans, peas, grains and seeds.

Partially alkaline foods

1. Fresh raw milk and curd.
2. Soaked nuts and seeds.
3. Fresh nuts - Almonds, Coconut, Brazil nuts.
4. Fresh green beans, peas, corn & millet.

Some useful notes

1. It can be seen from the table ahead that wholemeal wheat flour, unpolished rice and such other cereals in their more or less natural forms are only mildly acid-genic but processing or refining them makes them much more acidic in effect.

2. It can be seen that almost all cereals, pulses, all types of meats, egg, fish are acidic in nature while almost all fruits and vegetables are alkaline in nature.

3. All citrus foods (lemon, orange etc.) may initially appear acidic in nature but their ultimate effect in the body is alkaline. That is why they are classified as alkaline foods.

4. Legumes, beans being protinous foods, come under the category of acidic foods but when converted into sprouts, they turn more alkaline and less acidic.

5. There remains some doubt among people whether milk is acidic or alkaline in nature. In this connection, it is to be noted that fresh raw unboiled milk is alkaline in nature while boiled and heated milk is acidic. Various products derived from milk, e.g. cheese, butter, etc., are also acidic in nature.

6. It can be seen that among nuts, peanuts are most acid-genic while almonds are least acid-genic. Coconut, on the other hand, is alkaline in nature.

Relative Acidity and Alkalinity of Foods

Alkali-Genic Foods			
Food	Alkali-genic effect in percent	Food	Alkali-genic effect in percent
Fruits		**Vegetables, Tubers and Roots**	
Figs (Fresh)	27.81	Spinach	28.01
Raisins	15.10	Suva Plants	18.36
Grapes	7.15	Leafy Salad Plants	14.12
Sugar-cane	14.57	Cucumbers	13.50
		Beetroots	11.37
Tomatoes	13.67	Turnips	10.80
Lemons	9.90	Sweet Potatoes (Yams)	10.31
Oranges	9.61	Radishes	6.05
Plums	5.80	Potatoes	5.90
Dates	5.50	Peas (fresh)	5.15
		Cabbage	4.02
Peaches	5.40	Cauliflower	3.04
Apricots (fresh)	4.79	Onions	1.09
Bananas	4.38	Pumpkin	0.28
		Carrot	15.10
Pomegranates	4.15	**Milk**	
Coconuts	4.09	Skimmed Milk	4.89
Pineapples	3.59	Cream	2.66
Pears	3.26	Human Milk	2.55
		Cow's Milk	1.69
Watermelons	1.83	Butter Milk	1.31
Apples	1.38	Goat's Milk	0.25

Contd.

Acid Genic Foods			
Food	Acid-genic effect in percent	Food	Acid-genic effect in percent
Cereals		**Foods of Animal Origin (Excluding Milk)**	
Rice (polished)	17.96		
Rice (unpolished)	3.68		
Bread	10.99	Yolk of Egg	51.83
Barley	10.58	White of Egg	11.61
White Flour (Maida)	8.32	Egg	11.61
Maize	5.37	Beef	38.61
Wheat (Whole)	2.66	Chicken	24.32
		Goat's	20.30
Pulses and Legumes		Fish	19.52
All pulses and legumes are acid-genic		Pork	12.47
		Milk Products	
Nuts		Cheese	17.49
Peanuts	16.39	Butter	4.33
Walnuts	9.22	**Bakery Products**	
Almonds	2.19	Cake	12.31
		Chocolate	17.51

✿✿✿

Fibre-Less Foods

B efore we discuss about the harms caused by fibreless foods, we should first know something about the fibres and their role in the body.

What is fibre

Dietary fibres are the parts of plant foods which are resistant to digestion in human digestive tract. These are also called roughage and are mainly the skins and fibrous part of vegetables and fruits. Fibre comes from substances which make up the cell walls of plants.

Types of fibres

There are two types of fibres - soluble and insoluble.

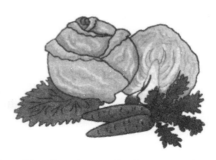

i.   **Soluble fibres:** They are soluble in water and become sticky in consistency. Examples include:

  – **Pectins** found in fruits (Apple, Banana), legumes (or pulses), nuts, some vegetables (carrot, potato), oat bran, barley, isabgol.

  – **Gums** such as guar or carageenam - found in algae, seaweeds and the cluster bean (guar ki phali).

  – **Mucilages** found in plant seeds and certain plant secretions.

ii. **Insoluble fibres:** They pass through the digestive tract largely unchanged except for being broken into smaller pieces by chewing. Examples include

- **Cellulose** which gives plant wall stability and structure and is found in bran, whole grains and vegetables.
- **Hemicellulose** is found in vegetables, fruits, nuts and whole grains.
- **Lignin**: a wood-like substance found in bran, fruit skins, nuts and whole grains.

Benefits of fibres

1. **Dietary fibre reduces cholesterol and lowers B.P.:** Liver is the chief site of cholesterol synthesis in our body. A part of cholesterol synthesised by the liver gets incorporated into bile acids and bile salts. Bile is secreted in the gut to help digestion and absorption of fats. It is normally reabsorbed by intestines and taken up by liver after digestion of food. Dietary fibre (mainly soluble fibre) interrupts this cycle by dissolving bile salts in it and preventing reabsorption of bile salts from the gut. The latter are thus excreted with undigested food. Similarly soluble fibre also binds dietary cholesterol (cholesterol present in the diet) which is excreted out of body along with fibre. By enhancing cholesterol excretion, fibre reduces the availability of cholesterol in the liver for incorporation into cholesterol rich particles (lipoproteins) for release in the circulating blood. By lowering cholesterol in blood, fibre indirectly helps in lowering B.P.

2. **Fibre controls blood sugar levels:** Fibre lowers the rate of glucose absorption from the gut and lowers glucose level in blood and therefore aids in treating diabetes. Fibre helps in reducing insulin dosage administered to the diabetic patient.

3. **Fibre prevents constipation:** Fibre has a high water holding capacity. It helps to keep faeces softer and bulkier and food moves through the intestinal tract more quickly. This prevents constipation and reduces the risk of large bowel cancer.

4. **Fibre helps in weight reduction:** Fibre makes a person feel full even though it doesn't contribute calories. This is because one has to eat food more slowly because the food needs

more chewing. One will swallow more saliva also in the process to fill stomach. Furthermore, fibre delays the absorption of carbohydrates and fats and therefore has satiety value. On high fibre diet, one is less likely to overeat. Thus it helps in weight reduction. A high fibre diet is always a low fat diet and a high fat diet is always a low fibre diet.

5. **Fibre decreases toxicity:** Fibre helps in reducing toxicity since it binds with toxic substances present in food.

How much fibre should be taken

There is, as such, no strict recommended dietary allowance (RDA) for fibre intake. However, nutritionists generally recommend that an average healthy adult should consume 30-40 gms of fibre each day.

Excessive intake of fibres can be harmful

Too much of dietary fibre

i.   may produce intestinal gas and abdominal bloating. Very high fibre diets often cause gas formation.

ii.   may bind and interfere with intestinal absorption of minerals like iron, zinc etc.

iii. may result in diarrhoea.

iv.   may lead to intestinal blockage which may require surgery to open. This is more common among older people whose bowel function is already sluggish.

Common eatables having no fibre or low fibre

1. White bread
2. Clear soup
3. Patties
4. Cake
5. Potato chips
6. Suji

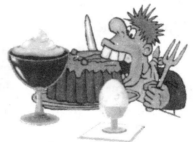

7. Noodles
8. Fruit juice
9. Meat, fish
10. Sugar
11. Egg
12. Pizza
13. Ice cream
14. Pastry
15. Polished rice (white)
16. Maida (White flour)
17. Vermicelli
18. Gulab Jamun
19. Milk
20. Fat (Oil, ghee, butter etc.)

Common eatables having good amount of fibre

Cereals: Wheat (whole), Oat, Maize, Bajra, Barley, Jowar, Dalia, Brown rice, Millet.

Pulses & Legumes: Kala chana, Rajmah, Kabuli chana, Soyabean, Redgram, Sprouted legumes or pulses, whole pulses (Whole Moong, Whole Urad, Whole Masoor etc.)

Vegetables: Beans, Peas, Carrot, Radish, Turnip, Beetroot, Cucumber, Cabbage, Lettuce, Spinach, Bhindi, Turai, Potato (with skin), Pumpkin.

Fruits: Guava, Apple, Banana, Grapes, Peaches, Pears, Figs, Prunes, Strawberry, Dry dates, Mango.

Opportunities for increasing fibre intake

1. Make a habit of taking a bowl of salad preferably mixed with sprouted pulses before every meal.
2. Consume fruits with edible peels.
3. Take 'Dalia' frequently in breakfast.
4. Take whole wheat chappati and whole wheat bread.

5. Use 'kala chana' in variety of ways e.g. missi roti, sprouts in salad, kala chana curry.

6. Fibre intake may be supplemented by use of isabgol, Oat bran, fenugreek (methi) seeds. Isabgol may be consumed by mixing it in a glass of water or milk or fruit juice or curd or lassi or sharbat. 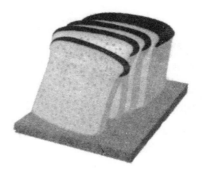 A teaspoon of fenugreek seeds with a glass of water before meals can also be very helpful.

7. Fruits should be eaten without peeling their skin which is the part most rich in fibre.

8. Consume potato along with its skin.

9. Limit the use of white bread, naan, roomali roti and other refined and processed food.

Harmful effects of low fibre or fibreless diet

A low or nil fibre diet may eventually lead to the following diseases in the body.

   i. Constipation

  ii. Colon cancer

 iii. High blood cholesterol and High B.P.

  iv. Obesity

   v. Haemorhoids

  vi. Many disorders of colon, rectum and intestines

 vii. Piles

Fibre Contents of Some Foods
(gm per 100 gm of food)

Bran	48	Whole wheat flour	11.7
Peas	7.7	Carrots	3.7
Cabbage	2.9	Banana	1.8
Plum	1.5	Apple	1.4
Tomatoes	1.4	Pear	2.4
Lemon	1.4	Peanut	3.1
Dates	3.9	Pulses/legumes	3 to 5
Fig	6.4	Guava	5.2
Coconut	6.6	Bitter gourd	
Pomegranate (Anar)	5.1	(Karela)	1.7

✿✿✿

Adulterated Foods

What is adulteration

Adulteration is defined as the process by which the quality or the nature of a given substance is reduced by the addition of a foreign or an inferior substance or the removal of a vital element.

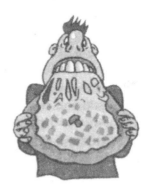

Mixing, substitution, abstraction, concealing the quality, misbranding and giving false levels are different forms of adulteration.

Types of Adulterants

i. **Intentional adulterants:** These include sand, marble chips, stone, mud, chalk powder, water to milk, harmful colours and mineral oils to edible oils.

ii. **Incidental adulterants:** These include pesticide residues, dropping of lizards, rodents and larva in food.

iii. **Metallic contamination:** It includes arsenic from pesticides, lead from water, mercury in industries etc.

Common adulterants used in various eatables

1. **Milk:** Addition of water, plain or contaminated, removal of partial or full cream, addition of starch, addition of paper pulp for forming a cream and addition of skimmed milk powder, addition of preservatives like boric acid, salicylic acid, borax (to prevent it from souring) are the common adulterants.

2. **Ghee:** This is adulterated by vanaspati and animal fats like pig's fat and boiled mashed potatoes. In order to improve the flavour of adulterated ghee, tributyrin is added.

3. **Pulses:** Arhar pulse is adulterated with lathyrus. Metallic yellow, a chemical substance, is added to old stock to improve its colour and appearance.

4. **Edible oil:** Cheaper and mineral oils are added. Argemone oil is mixed with mustard oil. Dyes are added to improve the yellowish colour of the oils.

5. **Tea and Coffee:** Tea is adulterated with used and exhausted tea leaves, dust, saw dust and black farm husk. Coffee powder is adulterated with roasted dates, tamarind seeds, added colour and chicory.

6. **Cereals:** Rice and wheat are mixed with stones, sand, grit and mud to increase the bulk. Besan is adulterated with lathyrus flour.

7. **Honey:** It is mixed with sugar and jaggery solution and is boiled with empty beehives.

Physical tests for detection of food adulterants

i. **Argemone seeds with mustard seeds:** Argemone seeds are black in colour but are not uniformly smooth and round.

ii. **Kesari Dal in Arhar:** Kesari dal is wedge shaped. Smaller one resembles masoor dal, the larger one is the size of arhar.

iii. **Iron fillings in Tea Leaves:** With the help of magnet, iron filling can be observed and removed physically.

iv. **Ergot seed in Bajra:** Ergot seeds are lighter than bajra and will float in water.

v. **Inorganic matter:** Like sand, gravels, dirt, pebbles can be observed and removed physically.

vi. **Coal tar dye:** May be present in roasted gram and tea leaves. Depositing the tea on a moistened blotting paper will show the presence of coal tar dye by spreading the colour on the blotting paper.

Simple laboratory chemical tests

i. **Metanil yellow in haldi powder or in gur:** In 2 gm of the sample, add 5 ml of alcohol. Shake and add a few drops of concentrated HCL. A pink colouration indicates presence of metanil yellow.

ii. **Addition of Starch:** (a) *To milk and butter:* Add a few drops of iodine solution to a small quantity of the sample. Formation of blue colour could indicate adulteration with starch.

(b) *To Coffee Powder:* Decolorise it by adding KMno4 solution. Then add drops of iodine solution. Blue colour formation indicates adulteration with starch.

iii. **Argemone oil in mustard oil:** Heat 5 ml of test sample with 5 ml of nitric acid for 2 to 3 minutes. A red colour will appear if argemone oil is present.

iv. **Artificial colour in red chillies:** Rub the chilli with a piece of cotton soaked in liquid paraffin. If the cotton extracts the red colour it shows adulteration.

✿✿✿

Foods Spoiled by Micro-Organisms

Foods are sometimes spoiled by the action of various microorganisms. Microorganisms include moulds, yeasts and bacteria. Some microorganisms exist in both forms, vegetative and spore. Spores are more resistant to destruction by heat or other agents than the vegetative form.

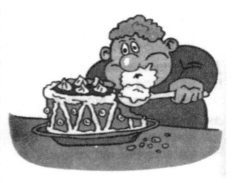

1. **Food spoilage by moulds:** Mould growth on foods with its cottony appearance makes food unfit for consumption. Moulds are most likely to develop in warm, damp and dark places between 25 to 30°C. Sunlight is an inhibitor for mould growth. Certain moulds in mild quantity are not harmful but a few can produce mycotoxins i.e. aflatoxins specially on groundnut, wheat, etc., if these are not dried as soon as they are harvested.

2. **Food spoilage by yeast:** Yeasts grow usually on food such as fruits which contain water and sugar. The typical musty smell of spoiled grapes is due to the growth of yeast. Yeast is reproduced by budding of cells. Yeast generally grows better in acid medium in the presence of sufficient oxygen between 25°C to 30°C. Yeast converts sugar of the fruit into alcohol and carbon dioxide. Honey, jams, jellies are contaminated by yeast.

3. **Food spoilage by Bacteria:** Bacteria is unicellular and much small in size. Aerobic bacteria grow in the presence of oxygen only while anaerobic bacteria grow in absence of oxygen. Bacteria usually spoil foods which are neutral in reaction such as milk, eggs, meats and vegetables.

4. **Action of enzymes:** Enzymes are organic catalysts produced by living cells. They are protein in nature and can act from 0°C to 60°C. Beyond a certain stage, enzymes themselves can render the fruits unfit for human consumption. For example, ripening of banana is caused by enzymes but beyond stage of ripening they spoil the banana.

Certain worms, bugs and fruit flies may also spoil the food.

Three conditions for spoilage of foods by micro-organisms

Microbes work best when the following conditions are present:

1. Presence of moisture   2. Presence of warmth
3. Presence of oxygen (air)

Ways to prevent decomposition of food by micro-organisms

There are normally four methods to keep food preserved for longer period of time.

1. Airtight/Vacuum packing (Eliminates air or oxygen)
2. Drying and dehydration (Removes moisture)
3. Refrigerating or freezing (Eliminates warmth)
4. Sterilisation by blanching or boiling (Kills bacteria, moulds and enzymes)

Anyone of these methods will break the chain of action causing food decay. Combining more than one method will further improve matters. The above techniques of preserving the foods belong to the subject of 'Food Preservation" which is a vast subject in itself and is outside the scope of this book.

✿✿✿

Chemical Additives in Foods

Introduction

The use of chemicals as food additives is an ancient practice, sodium chloride being the first to be used. Food additives are currently a part of our way of eating especially in the industrialised world.

According to one estimate, as many as 10,000 compounds or combinations of compounds may find their way into foods during processing, packaging or storage. These include unintentional additions also, e.g. residues of pesticides used to treat crops, minute amounts of drugs fed to animals (hormones, antibiotics) and chemicals that seep out of plastics and other packaging materials.

Why chemicals are added in food

Additives are generally used for solving complex problems of storing, cleaning, handling, heating and packaging commercially prepared foods. Some additives are merely used to preserve the natural colour of the foods (e.g., addition of nitrate to meat to preserve the pink colour). In brief these additives serve one or more of the following functions in foods:

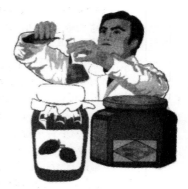

1. Preservatives
2. Buffers
3. Emulsifiers
4. Neutralising agents

5. Sequestering agents (or chelating agents)
6. Stabiliser
7. Anticaking agents
8. Flavouring and colouring agents

In addition, some additives are used as nutritional supplements to increase the nutritive value of foods, such as potassium iodide and vitamins. Before these chemicals are cleared for use, they are tested on experimental animals, one at a time.

Side effects of chemical additives

Humans ingest dozens of chemicals daily during the course of their lifetime. No one can say what overall effects these chemicals will have on the body; which chemicals are poisonous or carcinogenic by interacting with others; which are dissipated by the body and which are cumulative. For example, we have seen how the nitrates added to meat could transform into the carcinogenic nitrosamines by reacting with amino acids in the stomach. While most of these additives have been cleared as safe by the administrations of various countries, some continue to be controversial. Some examples are:

1. BHA (Butylated hydroxy anisole) and BHT (Butylated hydroxy toluene) as antioxidants

2. Red no.2 and no. 40 and Yellow no.5 as colouring agents

3. Carboxymethyl cellulose as a stabiliser

4. Aspartame and Sucralose as well as Saccharin as artificial sweeteners.

5. *Monosodium glutamate (MSG)*, also called *Chinese Salt*, is the best known flavour enhancer commercially used in oriental restaurants and in prepared foods. Earlier it was also used in baby foods but is now discontinued after studies showed that large amounts destroyed brain cells in young mice. Now MSG has been found to be responsible for the so-called Chinese restaurant syndrome which produces headaches, tightness in the chest and forearms accompanied by weakness and palpitations.

Common Chemical Additives in Food and Their Purpose

Class	Purpose	Examples	Uses
1. Acidulants	Appealing acid taste	Citric acid, Phosphoric acid, Malic acid, Furmaric acid, Tartaric acid, Lactic acid	Soft drinks, fruit juices, jams, soft drinks powders, etc.
2. Anticaking Compounds	Keeping powders crystalline and free-flowing by preventing absorption of moisture and caking	Calcium silicate, Magnesium silicate, Silica gel, Tricalcium Phosphate, Aluminium calcium silicate	Table salt, baking powder, malted milk powders
3. Antioxidants	Retard the oxidative breakdown of oils and fats and prevent rancidity	Butylated hydroxy anisole (BHA), Butylated hydroxy toluene (BHT), Propyl gallate	Cooking oils and fats, dehydrated foods
4. Artificial Sweeteners	Sweet taste	Saccharin, Calcium Cyclamate, Aspartame (banned)	Soft drinks, low calorie foods
5. Bleaching and maturing agents	Proper bleaching and ageing	Benzoyl Peroxide, Chlorine	Flour

Contd....

Class	Purpose	Examples	Uses
6. Colours	Pleasing appearance	Permitted synthetic colours, Cochineal, Caramel, Saffron, Turmeric	Butter, cheese, soft drinks, confectionery, jellies, etc.
7. Emulsifiers	Disperse one liquid in another	Lecithin, Saponins, Lipoproteins, Synthetic, glycerol, Esters of fatty acids, Polysorbates, Brominated vegetable oils (BVO)	Ice creams, confectionery coatings, cakes, soft drinks, etc.
8. Flavours	To provide flavour	Natural flavours like saffron, cinnamon, clove, pepper and fruit extracts, synthetic flavours like bezaldehyde, isoamyl acetate, Flavour enhancers like monosodium glutamate (Chinese salt)	All processed foods

Contd....

Class	Purpose	Examples	Uses
9. Leaven agents	Release of carbon dioxide from sodium bicarbonate (baking soda)	Phosphate, potassium acid tartrate, Sodium aluminium sulphate	Baking powder
10. Moisture retaining agents	Prevent escape of moisture	Sorbitol, Glycerol, Propylene glycol	Shredded coconut, candies
11. Additives for curing & ripening	Curing and ripening	Nitrate, Acetylene	Meat, fruits.
12. Preservatives	Controlling moulds, bacteria and other organisms	Calcium and Sodium propionates, sorbates, Sodium benzoate, Ethyl formate, Ethylene oxide, Propylene oxide, sodium sulphite and metabisulphite	Bread, cheese, jellies, cakes, fruit juice, yeast, etc.
13. Sequestrants	Improve the colour, flavour and texture of foods by tying up trace metals like iron, copper, zinc, etc.	Citric acid, Sodium Hexamitaphosphate, Sodium tripolyphosphate	All processed foods

Contd....

Class	Purpose	Examples	Uses
14. Stabilisers and thickeners	Texture and consistence	Gum arabic, Sodium carboxy-methyl cellulose, Gelatin, Agar, etc.	Syrups, gravies, chocolate milk, icings, cheese spreads, etc.
15. Nutrients	Replace vitamins and minerals lost in processing or supplement those not present	B group vitamins, Beta carotene (Vit A), Vitamin E, Vitamin C, Vitamin A and D, Iodine, Iron, etc.	Flour, cereals, milk, beverages, processed fruits, etc.

✿✿✿

Pesticides and Foods

Introduction

Pesticides are poisonous chemical substances which are sprayed over crop plants to protect them from pests (harmful small animals) and diseases. These include insecticides, fungicides, herbicides, rodenticides and weedicides.

The earliest chemical pesticides were nicotine, rotenone and pyrethrum from plant sources. The first synthetic pesticide was Paris Green - copper acetoarsenate - an inorganic compound. Other inorganic pesticides include lead arsenate, lime sulphur and fluorides.

D.D.T. and B.H.C. are some of the common pesticides used today. These pesticides are chlorinated hydrocarbons (Chlorine containing hydrocarbons) which are very toxic or poisonous. It has been found that urban people (city people) have damaging amount of pesticides like D.D.T. concentrated in their bodies.

The total amount of pesticides applied world wide is currently put at 2.5 million tones. Of this 50-60 per cent are herbicides, 20-30 per cent insecticides and 10-20 per cent fungicides.

Types of Pesticides

1. **Organochloro insecticides:** The first synthetic organic pesticide DDT (dichlorodiphenyltrichloroethane) was introduced in 1939. This was followed by other organochloro insecticides like Aldrin, BHC, Dieldrin and Heptachlor. The hazard associated with the use of Organochloro insecticides were realised when scientists discovered residues of these compounds building up in the fatty tissues of animals

and even humans. According to one report in 1970, the human fat from residents of New Delhi contained as much as 26 ppm, the highest in the world at that time. Their residues persist in the environment for long periods extending upto a few years causing adverse health effects like cancer.

2. **Organophosphates:** Organophosphates were introduced in 1930. These include Parathion, Malathion, Ronnel, Methoate and several others. Unlike organochloro compounds, these chemicals break down quickly when exposed to weather. But they are more poisonous to mammals than the organochlorines and have to be handled carefully.

3. **Carbamates:** A third class of insecticides, the carbamates, contain one or more amino groups. They do not leave harmful deposits on food. But some carbamates are harmful to warm-blooded animals. Carbaryl is a general purpose carbamate insecticide. Aldicarb is the most toxic carbamate.

4. **Pyrethroids:** A new class of insecticides called pyrethroids was introduced in 1970. These chemicals are similar to pyrethrum, a natural insecticide, but do not break down as quickly as the natural product. They attack the nervous system. They are not toxic to mammals but are lethal to fish. For this reason their use in steams, rivers and lakes has to be strictly controlled.

Ways of entry of pesticides in our bodies

The poisonous pesticides can enter our body in the following ways:

1. The pesticides enter our body directly when we don't wash the fruits and vegetables properly before eating them, on which pesticides had been sprayed in the fields.

2. When excessive pesticides are sprayed over the crops during their growth, then some of the pesticides goes inside the fruit (or grains etc.) of the crop and becomes a part of it. When men and animals eat such contaminated fruits or grains etc., then the pesticides enter their body and do the damage.

3. Pesticides which are sprayed over crop plants to protect them mix up with the soil and water. From soil and water, these pesticides are absorbed by the growing plants along with water and other minerals. When they are eaten, these chemical pesticides go into the bodies of animals and human beings.

4. Some of the chemical substances used on crop plants get washed down into the ponds, lakes, rivers and underground water bodies. Drinking of such contaminated water or eating the fish grown in such water also leads to the entry of these chemicals inside the human body.

Gradual build up of pesticides in food chain

Pesticides enter the food chain at the plants level. When the man and other animals eat these plants or their products like food grains, these poisonous chemical substances get transferred to their bodies. These harmful chemicals get concentrated at each successive higher level in food chain. Let us consider the following food chain for better understanding:

Grass → Sheep or Goat →Man

In this food chain, grass absorbs harmful chemicals from the soil. The sheep or goat receives these chemicals when they eat grass. When man drinks the milk of sheep or goat or when man eats the meat of sheep or goat, then these harmful chemicals present in the milk or meat of sheep or goat get transferred to his body and start accumulating there.

It has been found by experiments that the harmful chemical substances present in soil and water (due to spraying of pesticides) get concentrated at each successive trophic level (Plants → animals → man) with the result that the creature occurring at the highest trophic level in the food chain (e.g. man) has the maximum quantity of harmful chemicals in it. For example, water in a pond, lake or river has been found to contain only a small amount of .02 ppm (.02 parts per million) of the harmful chemicals in it. The algae and the protozoa which utilise this

110

water contain a higher proportion of 5 ppm of the harmful chemicals. The fish which feeds on these organisms has still higher amount of 240 ppm of these chemicals, and the birds and human beings which eat these fish have been found to contain as much as 1600 ppm of the harmful chemical substances in their bodies. This can be represented as

Water $\rightarrow$ Algae & Protozoa $\rightarrow$ Fish $\rightarrow$ Birds & Man

.02 ppm   5 ppm   240 ppm   1600 ppm

of chemicals   of chemicals   of chemicals   of chemicals

It has been found that the amount of poisonous chemical substances accumulated in human bodies is higher than that of other organisms which are lower in the food chain. For example, the concentration of harmful chemical called DDT is maximum in human bodies.

Harmful effects of pesticides on living beings

According to one report, only 10 per cent of the 35,000 pesticides introduced since 1945 have been tested for potential health effects. Exposure to these pesticides as well as their unregulated use is causing environmental health problems of serious dimensions. Annually about 0.5 million people are subjected to pesticide poisoning while deaths number 10,000 worldwide. According to one observer, in China there were people working in clouds of pesticides all the time and they were using the dirtiest possible pesticides. Such scenarios are very common in all developing countries. In fact, quite a large number of pesticides like the organochloro pesticides which are banned in developed countries are still widely used in developing countries because they are relatively cheap and easily available. The following are some of the detrimental effects from the use of various pesticides:

1. Many domestic animals are poisoned due to ingestion of pesticides and therefore significant quantities of meat and milk obtained through them are also contaminated by the pesticides.

2. When pesticides are applied to crops, natural enemies that are important for controlling some pests (e.g. birds) are frequently destroyed. This causes outbursts of pests that have to be controlled with additional applications of pesticides.

3. The development of pesticide-resistant pest population is proving to be a great problem. Where this occurs, additional treatment and sometimes stronger pesticides become necessary to kill these pests.

4. Large number of honey bees and wild bees are poisoned by pesticides resulting in honey losses and reduced pollination.

5. Some pesticides, especially when applied through aerial spray (e.g., from aircraft) and during periods of strong wind, drift into adjacent agricultural land and destroy the crops.

6. Significant losses of fisheries and wildlife occur from pesticide use.

7. Pesticides cause destruction of soil, invertebrates (e.g., earthworm), microflora and microfauna.

8. Pesticides cause chronic health problems such as allergies or diseases like cancer.

9. Pesticides cause ground water contamination. It is reported that 10.4 percent of US community water supply wells and 4.2 per cent of US domestic water supply wells contain detectable levels of pesticides.

Some recommendations

Although there is no way one can escape fully from the effect of chemicals and pesticides used in food but following measures will help to some extent in reducing their harmful effects:

1. Wash all fruits and vegetables in plenty of water before eating, specially where skin is also to be eaten.

2. Keep the food grains, fruits and vegetables for sometime in sunshine. This will dilute the effect of chemicals/pesticides to some extent.

3. For eating root vegetables in raw form (e.g. Carrot, Radish, Lettuce etc.) skin should be preferably peeled off to ward off the effect of pesticides. Leafy vegetables should preferably be eaten after boiling and not eaten raw for reduced ingestion of pesticides sprayed over them in the field.

ooo

Wrong Food
Combinations

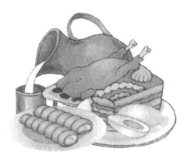

S ometimes you may be eating best foods but due to wrong combination these become harmful to us rather than beneficial. Hence it is desirable that one should understand the laws of food combination and their scientific basis.

When one eats an incompatible combination of foods, nature flashes a distress signal in the form of a belch (this also happens when one overeats). We should learn to heed this little warning of nature. In case one doesn't heed this warning and continues overeating and taking wrong combinations of foods, then following disorders may immediately follow:

1. Vomiting
2. Loose motion or diarrhoea
3. Indigestion of some foods which may be found in stools

Acid and other waste products of protein indigestion and putrefaction are easily identified in the urine. Scientifically they belong to the group of phenyls, skatoles, indoxyl-sulphuric acids, uric acid and toxic amines. Often they are eliminated vicariously through the mucous membranes or by diffusion into the spinal fluid.

Below are given some laws for right and wrong food combinations.

1. Milk shouldn't be combined with any other food. It should be taken alone

Milk never combines well with any other food. Milk is a complete and concentrated food in itself. It requires full digestive process of its own kind. No other concentrated food like meat, eggs, cereals, pulses, nuts, roots or fruits should be eaten with it. Milk is a totally different protein than other concentrated proteins like meat, eggs, nuts, etc. Milk doesn't digest in stomach but in duodenum hence in the presence of milk, stomach doesn't respond with its secretion. Milk prevents insalivation also, creating problems for digestion of starchy foods. Further being liquid, it can't go efficiently with any other food. This prevent the digestion of other foods taken along with milk. One should eat solid food and take milk separately.

Due to its fat and protein contents, on reaching the stomach, milk coagulates to form curd. This curd tends to gather around the particles of the other foods in the stomach thus insulating them against the gastric juices. This prevents their digestion until the milk curd is digested.

Combination of milk with other foods is one of the major causes of indigestion. However combination of milk with light snacks, e.g. biscuits, etc., is tolerable.

2. Starches and proteins shouldn't be taken together

All starches are digested in an alkaline media. But proteins are digested in acid media. When starches after mixing with salivary enzymes in the mouth, pause on to stomach with the proteins, heavy hydrochloric acid is poured out from the stomach to digest protein and starch digestion comes to an abrupt halt. Starches are forced to remain in the stomach until protein digestion is completed. By the time it reaches small intestine without full digestion it is already fermented due to long retainment in stomach. This great amount of undigested starches are found in stool.

It is not only starch that remains undigested but protein also remains undigested. The acid and alkali both contrast and neutralise each other inhibiting the digestive process of starch and protein.

If at all, you have to eat starches and proteins together, eat protein first and after 20-30 minutes follow the starch so that starch digestion doesn't come to complete halt in stomach. But nevertheless it is not an ideal combination.

From this angle roti-dal, rice with milk (Kheer), rice with fish, egg with bread, roti or rice and meat etc., are not ideal combinations. But it has been observed that since centuries we have been taking such combinations, our digestive system can well tolerate these combinations without any untoward effect. However, carbohydrates and proteins both can be eaten separately with vegetables liberally. From this angle Chapati eaten with cooked vegetables, Sprouts (proteins) taken with vegetable salad, Boiled potato (starch) taken with vegetable salad are good combinations.

3. Fruits and sugars shouldn't be combined with other solid foods, they should be taken alone

All sugars e.g., white sugar, syrup, jaggery, sweet fruit, honey etc., taken with protein, starches and fats hinder their digestion. Sugars undergo practically no digestion in mouth and stomach. They are primarily digested in the intestines. If taken alone, they are not held in the stomach for long but are quickly sent into the intestine. When eaten with other foods, either protein or starches or fats, they are held up in the stomach for a prolonged period awaiting the digestion of other foods and undergo fermentation. Fruits and sugar as a law, ferment with all solid foods and milk. Sugar is an acidic food. The fermentation of the sugar leads to further multiplication of the problems like acidity and indigestion.

If at all it is required to eat sweet things with other foods, it is preferable to eat the sweet thing sometime before the solid food is taken.

From this angle all those items in which sugar is mixed e.g., sweet curd, sweet lassi, sweet milk, ice-cream, kheer, sweet milk are not desirable.

4. Proteins shouldn't be taken along with acid or sour foods

Fruit acids (or any other acid like drug acids) interfere in gastric digestion of proteins either by destroying the pepsin or by inhibiting hydrochloric acid secretion. Gastric juices are not poured out in the presence of acidic or sour foods in the stomach. This seriously hinders protein digestion and this results in putrefaction.

Acid fruits are: Lemons, grapes, oranges, plums, prunes, sweet lemon (mosambi) strawerry, blackberry, malta, pineapples, pomegranates, tomato, tamarind etc.

Since curd is also acidic in nature so it should also be avoided taking with 'Dal' etc. From this angle, sprinkling lemon or putting tomatoes in cooked pulse (or Dal) is also not a good practice.

5. Don't take different kinds of proteins at the same time

Two proteins of different characters and different compositions call for different modifications of the digestive secretions and different timings of secretions in order to digest them efficiently. For example, the strongest juices are poured out upon milk in the last hours of digestion while in case of flesh, it is in the first hour of digestion. Similarly eggs receive the strongest secretion at a different time compared to that received by either flesh or milk. It is impossible to meet the requirement of two different proteins at the same meal. Two kinds of flesh or nuts or pulses may be taken together but not with totally different protein group. For example, nuts can be eaten with different nuts and flesh with different flesh.

From this angle 'Kadhi', 'Dahi vada', cheese omelette, paneer pakora, milk and nut-kheer are not ideal combinations. To conclude, take one concentrated protein at a meal otherwise indigestion of proteins may result.

6. Combination of curd with foods

Curd shouldn't be taken with

    i.   Starches (cereals like wheat, rice, potatoes, sago, etc.)

    ii. Proteins (nuts, legumes, beans, meat, fish, egg, etc.)

    iii. Sugars (white sugar, fruits, syrup and honey)

However, curd can be taken with raw and cooked vegetables. From this angle curd can be mixed in salad. Curd taken alone and without anything mixed in it is best.

7. Salt shouldn't be mixed in Salad'

This is because salt leaches water from salad which comes out along with nutrients. Thus salad loses its full benefits.

8. Carbohydrates shouldn't be taken with acid or sour fruits

This is because the sour or acid fruits deactivate the action of saliva which is necessary for digestion of carbohydrates. List of sour or acid fruits is already given in point no.4. Since curd is also acidic in nature so it should also be avoided taking with carbohydrates.

9. Avoid eating Acid fruits with sweet fruits

Acid fruits slow down the quick digestion of the sugars of sweet fruits leading to fermentation. Examples of sweet fruits are banana, papaya, dates, figs, sugarcane, chikoos, raisin, sweet berry, etc. However, acid fruits can be taken or mixed with vegetable/salad. According to this, sprinkling 'Neembu' (lemon) over salad and taking tomato in salad is perfectly O.K.

10. Avoid eating fats with proteins

Fat depresses the action of the gastric glands and inhibits the release of proper gastric juices which are required for protein digestion. It lowers entire digestive tone by more than 50%. Fat insulated foods remain for long time in digestive process demanding overactivity and strain. Heated and fried fats are more dangerous.

This is the reason why dairy products don't digest as quickly as other protein foods because these foods contain enough fat to inhibit gastric secretions for a longer time and so they have delayed digestion. From this consideration putting too much ghee in 'Dal' or frying 'Dal' in ghee is not a very good practice.

Unlike proteins, combination of carbohydrates with fats is tolerable. Hence a little 'ghee' applied on 'roti' during eating and taking bread butter as breakfast snack is acceptable.

11. Don't combine tea, coffee, alcohol and soft drinks with solid foods

These beverages severely restrict the proper gastric secretions and therefore the normal digestion is hindered.

12. Some miscellaneous recommendations

  i. Don't take pulpy (गूदे वाले) and juicy fruits together e.g. Banana and orange, apple and mosambi)

  ii. Don't take sugar or sweets with sweet fruits.

 iii. Don't take fruits and vegetables together.

  iv. Water shouldn't be drunk after eating cucumber, watermelon and Papaya.

  v. Milk and curd shouldn't be taken together.

  vi. Milk shouldn't be taken after eating radish.

 vii. Water shouldn't be drunk immediately after taking rice. It may lead to coughing.

Foods to be consumed alone

1. Milk: It is already explained earlier.

2. Melons: Melons ('Kharbooja', 'Tarbooj') digest quickly than other foods and may ferment even with fruits sometimes. Being sweet fruits, they can be occasionally tolerated with sweet fruits but not with acid and sour fruits.

3. Liquids: As a law, no liquid should be taken with solids. Liquid tends to pass away immediately into the intestines taking away all the digestive enzymes thus inhibiting the digestion.

Liquids should be taken at least 20 minutes prior to meal and not immediately after or along with meal but can be taken one hour after meal.

4. **Fruits:** should be taken alone and at least half an hour before meal but never with or immediately after meals. Reason is already explained at relevant place.

5. **Sugars:** All sugary products like sweets, sugary drinks and beverages should be taken alone preferably 30 minutes before the meals but shouldn't be taken with or immediately after meals.

6. **Fruit juices:** All fruit juices are passed faster than fruits into the intestine. Its stagnation with solids leads to their fermentation. Hence they should be taken alone.

7. **Acid fruits:** As already explained, acid fruits retard protein and starch digestion and will also ferment when taken with solid foods because of delayed absorption. Hence they should be taken alone on empty stomach. However, they can be taken before meal with salad and vegetables but should be avoided with sweet fruits.

8. **Milk products:** Like milk, various milk products e.g. Yoghurt/curd, Ice cream, Rabri, Kulfi, Lassi, Buttermilk should also be consumed alone.

Tolerable combination of foods

Please note that what is given in this chapter are ideal combinations of foods. But it has been observed over years of experience that there are some combinations, which although not ideal, can be tolerated by our digestive system without any untoward effect on our health provided our digestive system is not weak or diseased. Some of such combinations are listed as follows.

1. Cereals+Pulses e.g. Roti+Dal, Rice+Dal
2. Cereals+Buttermilk or curd
3. Kheer (Rice+Milk)
4. Rice with fish, egg cury, meat
5. Bread+Egg omelette
6. Kadhi, Dahi vada
7. Ghee with Dal
8. Lemon+Sprout, Tomato+Sprouts

9. Sweet fruits+Acid fruits
10. Melons+Sweet fruits
11. Egg+Milk
12. Nuts+Milk
13. Milk+Bread sandwich
14. Banana+Milk
15. Mango+Milk
16. Jalebi+Milk
17. Curd+Rice
18. Curd+Banana

You can also make any number of such tolerable combinations depending on your own experience with them. I may also inform the readers that all these theories of food combinations are under continuous research and no final words with a rigid stand can be said about them. Intellectuals may further probe in these areas taking the matter of this chapter as some sort of reference or rough guidelines.

Four most important points to improve your digestion

1. Eat only when you are hungry. Body can tolerate even wrong combination of foods in strong genuine hunger.

2. Strengthen your digestive system by various exercises, etc. Strong digestive system can easily tolerate occasional wrong combination of foods taken.

3. Take one type of food or lesser varieties of food at a time. More variety of food puts great strain on digestive system since body can handle one food at a time more smoothly. It has no provision to secrete many juices and digest different foods at one time. Hence many variety of foods taken at a time result in delayed, imperfect digestion and fermentation and putrefaction.

4. Consume natural live raw foods to the maximum (e.g., fruits, vegetables, sprouts, nuts, etc.)

✿✿✿

Some Facts about Milk

Traditionally milk has always been considered a complete and perfect food. However, despite its several benefits, many people have been reporting several reactions to taking milk such as

1. Stomach and other cramps

2. Diarrhoea or loose stools

3. Nausea and sometimes vomiting

4. Flatulence (gas)

5. Bloating

6. Nasal symptoms and lot of mucous formation

7. Allergy of various kinds

Noticing these reactions, many researches have been done over milk and its utility and some startling revelations have come out which point out towards some harmful aspects of usage of animal milk by man. I would like to present a gist of these researches to the readers for their scientific understanding about the properties and usage of milk.

New scientific researches have drawn two important conclusions about the usage of milk by human beings -

1. Each species' milk is most suitable only for species of that nature. Every mammal's milk is designed and

intended for the development of its young ones. Except human beings no animal drinks the milk of any other animal.

From this consideration, the best milk for a human being is the milk of his own mother. The composition of milk of every species is different and is suited to body requirement of its own species only.

2. The greatest requirement of milk is only during the infancy when the infant is not able to take any other food. Milk is not meant for lifelong use. No animal except man takes milk lifelong.

    From this consideration, the usage of milk should considerably reduce in adulthood. Its greatest requirement is for the young one upto 3-4 years, till teeth are evolved for independent mastication and he is able to digest solid foods properly. Infact, nature has automatically provided the required quantity and quality of milk in mother's breasts as is needed by an infant to grow properly.

We can now elaborate on the properties of milk to make the above mentioned two points more clear to the readers from scientific angle.

1. **Protein in milk:** Cow's milk has 3 times more proteins and almost 4 times more calcium. This is because the growth rate of calves is much more than human infants. Cow's milk contains fast growing steroids and hormones. If we drink this milk with such constituents in it meant for the structure and growth of a calf, it is bound to create imbalance in our body.

    Moreover, cow's milk proteins are more coarser while mother's milk proteins are much finer. A child fed on cow's milk forms cheese clumps in the stomach and when the child vomits, he expels cheese. On the other hand, a child fed on mother's milk vomits only fine flakes.

    More protein means more acidity in the body because protein is an acidic food and to neutralise this acid,

123

calcium is leached out from bones and teeth and they become weak. Further, excess protein places additional burden on the kidneys leading to their premature degeneration due to overwork.

About 1.2% of breast milk is protein. This protein is made up of curd protein (casein) and whey proteins (lactoalbumin and lactoglobulin). Cow's milk has 3.3% protein and this extra is composed of 6 times as much casein as there is in breast milk.

When milk enters a baby's stomach, it is turned into curds and whey. The curds are made of casein. The curds of cow's milk are much bulkier and tough than those of breast milk because of higher amount of casein and sometimes lead to indigestion in some babies. Many people add water in milk to dilute this tough indigestible casein.

Breast milk protein forms finely separated curds in the stomach which then passes quickly and easily into the small intestine where they are easily broken down. This is why stomach of a breast fed baby empties more quickly than that of a bottle fed baby and baby gets hungry more quickly and needs frequent feeds. Cow's milk curds stay in the stomach for about 4 hours.

A baby uses only about half the protein available in cow's milk while a breast fed baby uses all the protein with virtually no wastage. Unused protein in cow's milk is partly passed out in the stools (which makes a bottle fed baby's stools bulkier than a breast fed baby's) and partly broken down before being excreted by the kidneys in the urine.

The lactoglobulin fraction of milk protein contains highly specialised proteins - the immunoglobulins (IgA, IgD, IgE, IgG and IgM). These carry the antibodies against disease. For years it was thought that a baby only obtained antibodies from its mother before birth across the placenta and that none were given via breast milk. We now know that babies continue to receive these essential antibodies from their mother's milk. *Colostrum* - a special sort of milk produced in the first few days after birth contains large amount of lactoglobulin, so colostrum is vitally important for the future health of the baby. Mature breast milk also contains antibodies but in smaller amounts. These milk antibodies are similar to those which the mother has in her blood and protect the baby against bacterial and viral illnesses from which the mother has suffered or has been immunised against. Among the illnesses that a baby can be protected, in this way, are tetanus, whooping cough, pneumonia, diptheria, E. Coli, Gastroenteritis, typhoid, dysentery, flu and various other viral illnesses including Polio. Later, a baby will manufacture his own antibodies in response to infection or immunisation. Immunoglobulin A (IgA) in the mother's colostrum and milk coats the lining of the baby's gut in the first few days after birth and prevents many infective organisms and other large protein molecules from entering the baby's bloodstream.

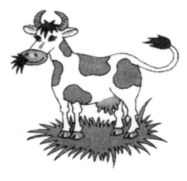

Cow's milk contains antibodies too but these are antibodies against cow's diseases, not human ones. Further lactoglobulin (together with lactogerrin, another anti-infective agent) is altered to such an extent by heating of cow's milk that it loses its antibody activity. That is why problems of gastro-enteritis are more with ingestion of cow's milk.

Besides protein in milk, there are free amino acids and the proportions of these differ in human and cow's milk. Breast milk contains more *cystine* compared with cow's milk which contains more *methionine*. This point is especially important for premature babies because they are incapable of using methionine until they become more mature.

2. **Fats in milk:** Fat present in cow's/buffalo's milk is present more in saturated form which increases cholesterol while breast milk contains a higher percentage of unsaturated fat.

Fats are split into simpler fatty acids in the gut by naturally occurring enzymes called lipases. The digestion of cow's milk fat by lipase leads to release of a fatty acid called *palmitic acid* which combines with calcium in the gut and is passed out in the stools, so robbing the body of calcium. In human milk, palmitic acid is built into the fat particles in such a way that when fat is digested by lipase, the acid is not released as a free fatty acid but is absorbed in the bloodstream together with part of the broken down fat particle. In this way calcium is not lost. Human milk contains some lipase of its own unlike cow's milk which relies solely on lipase in the body's intestine for its digestion. The fat in breast milk starts getting digested by the milk lipase even before it reaches the gut.

It is seen that when a breast fed baby vomits, there is no unpleasant smell whereas a bottle fed baby's vomit has a characteristic foul, sour smell. The difference is due to the presence of a fatty acid called butyric acid in cow's milk which smells nasty when partially digested.

3. **Calcium in milk:** Human beings absorb less calcium from a high calcium cow's milk than from the lower calcium mother's milk. It is not the quantity that counts but calcium is absorbed depending on the ratio of calcium and phosphorus in the milk which is inappropriate in cow's milk for absorption of calcium by human body.

Inappropriate absorption of calcium increases problem of acidity and tooth decay. Unfunctional calcium either gets deposited on some soft tissues in the form of plaque or is excreted in urine. Kidneys are overburdened in this process.

4. **Carbohydrates in milk:** Mother's milk has double the carbohydrate than found in cow's milk. So cow's milk is deficient in this nutrient. This is why breast fed baby hesitates to accept the sweetless cow's milk. Cow's milk is

usually not fed pure but sometimes added with 1/3 or 1/2 water in it. This makes milk absolutely tasteless and sweetless. Artificial sugar is added in cow's milk to make it artificially sweetened. Thus white sugar is unnecessarily introduced to child's stomach. Excess sugar may harm his pancreas by stimulating the overflow of insulin too early in life.

Breast milk also contains some glucose and some other sugars which are completely absent or present in much lower quantities in cow's milk.

The bifidus factor (explained further) is another carbohydrate present in breast milk but virtually absent from cow's milk. This is a very valuable protective factor against infection in the gut.

5. **Minerals:** Whole cow's milk contains almost 4 times as many minerals as breast milk because of which baby's kidneys have to work hard.

Cow's milk has 6 times more phosphorous and 3 times more sodium than the mother's milk. These excess materials not needed by human body create waste matter in the body and more load on kidneys for excretion.

Iron is one mineral present in larger amount in breast milk (twice than cow's milk). Iron in breast milk is better absorbed into the bloodstream than the cow's milk. Certain substances such as Vit. C, E and copper help iron to be absorbed more efficiently which are present in higher amount in breast milk.

Comparison of Nutrients in Human and Cow's Milk (per 100 gm)

	Human milk	Cow's milk
Protein (gm)	1.2	4
Fat (gm)	4	3.5
Carbohydrate (gm)	9	4.9
Calcium (gm)	33	118
Phosphorous (gm)	18	97
Sodium (gm)	16	50

6. **Mucous formation:** There is 300% more casein in cow's milk than in mother's milk. This casein coagulates in the stomach and forms large, tough, difficult to digest curds. The by products of the bacterial decomposition of casein end up in thick rope like mucous that sticks to mucous membranes and clogs our bodies. Infact it has been found that cow's milk produces more mucous than any other food. Thick dense mucous clogs and irritates the body's entire respiratory system, coats the inside of the body and prevents the fluid operation of the system. It adheres to the lining of the intestines and prevents the absorption of nutrients from the body which results in lethargy and diseases. It places a tremendous burden on the eliminative system of the body.

7. **Animal's milk creates constipation:** In breast milk the proportion of water and other constituents are just right for baby while in cow's milk, proportion of liquid to solid is less which may aggravate the problem of dehydration. If a child is already dehydrated due to diarrhoea, vomiting or sweating, the problem becomes more acute.

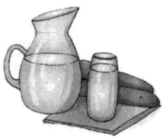

The stools of bottle fed babies contain less water than those of breast fed babies and this is one reason why they get constipated more often.

8. **Milk allergy:** Cow's milk has been often reported to produce allergy to many people in the form of diarrhoea, vomiting, colic, eczema, running nose, cough, wheezing etc. Infact many other illnesses are also caused by allergy to cow's milk protein. The protein most commonly involved is the B-lactoglobulin in cow's milk which is absent in breast milk. The reason for this is explained below.

Babies begin to make their own immunoglobulin A (IgA) after the first few weeks of life. Until they make enough, they need IgA from their mother's milk. Cow's milk IgA is no help as it is spoilt by heating. IgA is important in preventing allergic diseases because it forms a protective coating over the gut lining and not only fights infection but also stops infective organisms and large protein molecules leaking through the gut wall into the bloodstream.

In babies who are bottle fed there is no protective coating of IgA until the body makes enough of its own (in 3 months or so). Thus food proteins can leak into the blood stream through the gut wall and be taken to various body parts where they can set up an allergic response.

9. **Anti-infective factors:** We have already mentioned about antibodies in breast milk but there are other substances which also help fight infection in the baby and these are plentiful in breast milk than in cow's milk.

The very proportion of food substances in breast milk prevents the growth of certain organisms such as E. coli, dysentery and typhoid bacteria in the baby's gut. The high lactose, low phosphorus and low protein levels contribute to it.

The gut of baby contains thousands of tiny organisms. The organisms in the breast fed baby are members of the Lactobacillus bifidus family and are encouraged to grow by a special nitrogen containing sugar - the bifidus factor which is not present in cow's milk. The lactobacilli produce acetic and lactic acids which together prevent the growth of many disease producing organisms such as E. coli (a common cause of gastroenteritis), the dysentery bacillus and the yeasts.

An important anti-infective factor present in much greater amount in breast milk than in cow's milk is the protein lactoferrin. Together with one of the immunoglobulins (IgA) lactoferrin inhibits the growth of many organisms including E. coli, the yeasts and staphylococci by robbing them of the iron they need for growth.

Three more factors interact with each other to kill bacteria: *Lysozyme* (present in breast milk 300 times greater than cow's milk), Immunoglobulin A and a substance called complement. Lysozyme is present in other body secretions also, such as tears where it prevents infections of the eyes and eyelids.

Breast milk also contains an anti-staphylococcal factor, hydrogen peroxide and vitamin C which together kill bacteria such as E. coli. It contains an enzyme lactoperoxidase which inhibits the growth of bacteria and many live cells. These live cells are like white cells in the blood stream. Breast milk is a living fluid while cow's milk cells get killed by the time it reaches inside the baby because of the heating and other processes involved including the time factor.

The lymphoid cells in breast milk make IgA as well as an antiviral substance called *interferon*. These cells can also be absorbed from the gut into the bloodstream of the baby where they continue their work of making immunoglobulins. Other cells in breast milk are called *macrophages*. These are large cells which can actively engulf particles such as bacteria and also produce lactoferria, lysozyme and complement.

10. **Milk intolerance with growth:** There are two elements in milk that have to be broken down by the enzymes in the body - *Lactose* and *casein*. Lactose is broken down by the enzyme *lactase* and casein is broken down by the enzyme *renin*.

It is found that enzyme *lactase* is no longer (or very little) produced after the baby is weaned from its mother's milk between the age of two to four. By the age of three and four, renin is also almost nonexistent in the human digestive tract. This is how many people have acute reaction to milk including cramps, intestinal gas and diarrhoea. 'Lactose intolerance' in children and adults is nothing but inability to digest milk sugar (Lactose) due to deficiency of enzyme 'Lactase'. If a child below the age of four also show this intolerance because of hereditary/genetic reasons, then that

130

child can be given curd, paneer etc., to compensate for the requirement of milk.

This also proves that as we grow towards adulthood, nature wants us to drink less and less milk and take other things like fruits, vegetables, nuts, cereals & pulses, soups, coconut milk, soybean milk etc.

Milk products

Since what is true about milk is also more or less true about usage of various milk products, hence it will be worthwhile to mention about various milk products for reader's guidance.

1. **Cream:** It is the fat portion of milk. When milk is churned in centrifugal machine, cream is separated from the milk. If raw milk is kept in Refrigerator as such, layers of cream come up after sometime.

2. **Skimmed milk (or 'Sapratta' milk):** When cream is separated out from the milk, the remaining portion is skimmed milk or 'Sapratta'.

3. **Butter:** When cream is churned in a pan, butter (the fatty portion) is separated out as one product and 'mattha' (or butter milk) as other product. It can also be made from 'Malai' of milk as mentioned in (8).

4. **Buttermilk:** (Mattha or 'Chaj') is produced as explained in (3). It has no fat. It can also be made from 'Malai' of milk as mentioned in (8).

5. **Ghee:** When butter is heated, ghee is separated out.

6. **Curd:** When a little amount of curd is added to milk, whole of it gets converted into curd within 4 hours in summer and 12 hours in winter. When curd is added to milk, the lactobacillus bacteria (or lactic acid bacteria) present in it cause conversion of milk sugar called lactose into lactic acid (which is sour in taste) and thus convert milk into curd. By mixing curd in fatty or non-fatty milk, you can get the curd of corresponding nature (i.e. fatty curd or non-fatty curd). Curd is more easily digestible

131

than milk and curd bacteria keep the stomach and intestines in order.

7. **'Lassi':** It is made by churning 'curd' and converting it into liquid form by adding some water and adding sugar or salt in it.

8. **'Malai':** When milk is boiled, and it is allowed to cool, a crust formation takes place at the top of the milk which is called 'malai'. It contains major portion of fat of milk. When 'malai' is churned (after mixing little curd in it), 'Mattha' & butter get separated out.

   Note: Difference between 'Cream' & 'Malai' - Cream is obtained from Raw milk. Malai is obtained from boiled milk.

9. **'Rabri':** When milk is continued to boil, water present in it starts evaporating and milk is solidified to required consistency. Then sugar is added in it to make it 'Rabri'.

10. **'Khoya' or 'Mawa':** is like 'Rabri' except that solidification of milk is more in this case and moisture content is less.

11. **Paneer (Cheese):** When milk curdles by the use of some acid or vinegar then liquid gets separated out called 'whey' and remaining solid portion is 'Paneer'. In this process, milk protein 'casein' is coagulated and Paneer is obtained. Paneer has all the proteins and fats as that in the milk. Depending upon the use of fatty or non-fatty milk, we can make cheese having fat or fat free cheese. In market many types of processed cheese are available. They are made by adding different compounds and preservatives in soft cheese. Cheese is more acidic in nature.

12. **Whey:** It is the watery portion of milk after cheese is separated out.

13. **Kulfi:** It is made from 'Rabri' after freezing it.

14. **Pasteurised milk:** Normally if the fresh milk is not boiled for sometime, it gets spoiled. In the process of pasteurisation, milk is heated upto certain temperature and then suddenly cooled. Pasteurisation not only protects the milk from being spoiled but also kills the bacteria of tuberculosis, typhoid,

cholera, dysentery, etc. But with this process, many nutrients (like vitamins & enzymes) are destroyed and many chemical alterations take place. Also its value as a live food decreases. It is a law that any food when heated above blood temperature will start losing its nutritive value.

A few words about curd, buttermilk and whey

Among all the milk products, yoghurt, buttermilk and whey have a special place and carry some distinct benefits because of which they are normally recommended. Their salient features are as follows.

Yoghurt/Curd

1. Yoghurt is a useful source of calcium and phosphorus for strong bones and teeth. People who need calcium but can't drink milk because of lactose intolerance may take yoghurt.

2. It contains vitamin B_2 (riboflavin) which is needed to release energy from food and B_{12} for a healthy nervous system.

3. Live or fresh yoghurt discourages the proliferation of harmful bacteria and yeasts in the gut that lead to bowel infection.

4. It can help to relieve gastrointestinal disorders, diarrhoea and constipation. It can also reduce bad breath associated with some digestive disorders.

5. After a course of antibiotics, eating live yoghurt can restore the necessary intestinal bacteria destroyed by these drugs. It is to be noted that antibiotics not only destroy harmful bacteria but they simultaneously destroy useful bacteria residing in our gut which produce small amounts of some B vitamins and vitamin K for use by the body.

Buttermilk: Buttermilk is light, cooling and more easily digestible. The lactic acid of the buttermilk is a good food acid and is utilised by the body just as are the citric, malic and other acids found in fruits and some vegetables. The lactic acid also opposes intestinal putrefaction. In the presence

133

of this acid, germs which cause infections leading to diarrhoea and dysentery can't thrive. This acid makes buttermilk a natural laxative and stimulant of the colon. Free and regular use of buttermilk promotes longevity and prevents disorders of stomach and liver. A few caraway seeds in buttermilk first thing in the morning, relieve constipation with a certainty.

Whey is the water portion of milk after cheese is separated. It is rich in vitamins and contains milk sugar and much of the minerals. It is useful in jaundice and dysentery.

Conclusion

The purpose of this article is not to conclude that one shouldn't take milk at all. Purpose of this article is to stimulate the reader's mind to probe further in this area of interesting researches on milk and other foods and find their own conclusions instead of accepting blindly what has been said here.

Personally my conclusion so far is that one should definitely reduce animal milk's intake as one grows towards adulthood but not make it zero as milk definitely has some beneficial elements also along with the shortcomings as enumerated before. By taking less milk, one will be able to get those benefits and also avoid the shortcomings associated with it. But with reduction of milk, one should increase his intake of other healthier alternatives of foods e.g. fruits, vegetables, nuts, whole grained cereals & pulses, soyabean, coconut, soups etc.

✿✿✿

Miscellaneous Eatables and Their Harmful Ingredients

The description given below only gives the harmful elements contained in the following foods but it doesn't mean that they are totally harmful and shouldn't be taken at all. They have got some beneficial nutrients also. That's why their occasional use is permissible.

1. **Ice water (or chilled/refrigerated water):**

    1. Ice water impairs the functioning of the spleen and stomach. Therefore the digestion of food is hampered.

    2. Ice water or other drinks make the body and its joints stiff and aggravate arthritis and rheumatic problems. According to Ayurveda, it increases 'vayu' in the body.

    3. Ice creates inertia in the body.

2. **Soft drinks (or carbonated drinks or cola drinks):**

They are sweetened aerated drinks charged with CO_2 under pressure. The principal ingredients of soft drinks are:

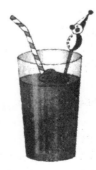

   i. Carbondioxide (CO_2)

   ii. Sugars

   iii. Citric acid (preservative)

   iv. Colouring agent

   v. Flavouring agent

   vi. Caffeine

   vii. Baking Soda (Sodium bicarbonate)

   viii. Phosphoric acid (Ethylene glycol)

   ix. Antifreeze compound

In addition they are ice cold also. It can be seen that most of these substances are harmful for the body. Unlike popular belief, I may clarify that these drinks are acidic (because of CO_2, sugar & citric acid) and not alkaline in nature. Only the soda contained in them produces a little alkaline effect. The only plus point with these drinks is that they help to replace lost fluid and energy very quickly after vigorous activity.

3. **Coco drinks:** Coco drinks (e.g., coca cola, pepsi, thumps up etc.) have a substance 'cocaine' in it in addition to other substances usually found in other soft drinks. Cocaine is obtained from coca leaf. *Cocaine is a stimulant and is addictive in nature* and comes under the category of 'Narcotic drugs'.

4. **Ice-cream:** The ice cream usually contains 20-25% cream and milk products, 15% sugar and sometimes egg and then lot of chemical additives as stabilisers, emulsifiers, buffers, synthetic colours, surfactants, artificial flavours and preservatives. Stabiliser is used in order to retain the smoothness of the ice-cream by preventing the formation of coarse ice crystals.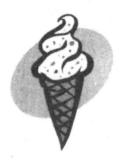

All these chemical additives are harmful and some of them, even cancer producing. Sugar, ice and saturated fat of milk further add to the harmful effects.

In ice creams prepared by local manufacturers without any control, lot of cheap chemicals are used and substandard materials in place of sugar and milk/cream are used which increase the damaging effect on the body further. The only benefits of Ice-cream are that most varieties contain vitamins A, B_2 & B_{12} plus they contain calcium.

5. **Cakes, Pastries, Cream roll:** The harmful ingredients in these are white flour (maida), white sugar, high saturated fat (Butter/cream/Dalda) and high dietary cholesterol (because of egg).

6. **Jams & Jellies:** The harmful ingredient in these substances is excess white sugar. Many jams contain natural organic compounds called *salicylates* and many cheaper brands contain artificial colours which may trigger allergies in some people.

7. **Biscuits (Cookies):** The harmful ingredients in these are

   (i) White flour (Maida)

   (ii) White sugar

   (iii) Saturated fat (Butter/hydrogenated fat)

   (iv) Artificial Flavours/essences

   The only advantage of biscuits are that they are convenient snack foods and rich source of carbohydrates. Now a days fibre-rich biscuits are also available.

8. **Patties, Samosa:** They are harmful mainly because of white flour (Maida), salt and excess oil/fat used for frying them.

9. **Namkeens, Chips:** They are harmful mainly because of salt and excess fat/oil used for frying them.

10. **Sweet meats:** The harmful substances in sweetmeats are mainly white sugar and cholesterol (since sweets are usually prepared in 'khoya' or 'paneer' which are milk products). Some sweets, e.g. 'Gulab Jamun' have additional disadvantage of being fried.

11. **Pizza, Bread, Bund, Burger:** The harmful elements in all these are mainly white flour (maida) and salt. Cheese spread on Pizza adds to saturated fat and cholesterol. Burger has an additional fried 'aloo tikki' in it.

12. **Pickles and chutneys:** Pickling is a traditional way of preserving fresh fruit and vegetables by discouraging the growth of microbes that would otherwise cause them to decompose. The food to be pickled is usually immersed in hot or cold vinegar and then the containers are sealed. Vinegar discourages the growth of harmful microbes and gives the food a tangy flavour. Salt is often mixed to reduce the moisture content. Thus sodium level of the food is much increased.

Many nutrients are lost in the pickling process although some vitamin C is retained. Sugar often added to chutneys and fruit chutneys may consist of as much as 50% sugar.

13. **Toffees, Candies:** Toffees contain mainly the following things - sugar, water, milk powder, glucose, white flour, artificial flavours/colouring agent.

The harmful ingredients in these are sugar, white flour and flavouring/colouring chemicals. Milk contributes to increase in cholesterol.

14. **Chocolate:** contains a substance 'cocoa' which is obtained from the ripe seeds of cocoa beans after they have been sweetened, dried, roasted and deprived of their shell. Cocoa is stimulating in nature and so causes all those harms which any other stimulant does. The stimulating principle in cocoa is 'theobromine'. Chocolate contains a substance 'Tyramine' which is alleged to trigger migraine attack.

Chocolate also contains caffeine, white sugar and artificial flavours which are harmful substances. Milk powder in chocolates contributes to increase in cholesterol level. Chocolate however contains some useful minerals like iron, magnesium and potassium.

15. **Sauce, Ketchup:** The harmful elements in these are excess sugar, salt, red chillies and chemical preservatives (citric acid etc.).

16. **Squashes:** The harmful elements are (i) Sugar (ii) Chemical preservatives (citric acid etc.). In case, ice is added in making 'sharbat' then it is another harmful ingredient.

17. **'Mathari' and Namakpara:** They have three harmful ingredients
    (i) White flour
    (ii) Salt
    (iii) Fried fat (these are fried in fat/oil)

18. **Tinned or canned foods:** The process of canning preserves foods by sealing them in air tight containers

and cooking them to a sufficiently high temperature to ensure that they are sterile. Because any microorganisms inside the container are killed and air is excluded, tinned foods will keep for a long time without deteriorating. However their disadvantages are:

 i. Many tinned foods are high in salt.
 ii. Colour, texture and taste of foods are altered.
 iii. Some nutrients are lost during heating (e.g. vit. B_1 & C). It is however observed that vit. A, D & riboflavin are retained.
 iv. Tinned food no more remains a live food. Its life energy or prana is lost in the process.

19. **Frozen foods:** Keeping foods at or below-18°C (0°F) significantly slows down spoilage. The major losses are the water soluble vitamins (B & C) from vegetables & fruits which leach out during blanching which is done before freezing the food. Blanching (exposure of food to very high heat) is done to halt the action of enzymes within the food and to prevent spoilage. Some food don't freeze well and freezing changes the structure of many fruits. Infact frozen food is not a live food. Its life energy or prana is lost.

20. **Pakoras:** Its main disadvantages are its salt content and excess fat/oil used for frying it in Bengal gram flour ('Besan').

21. **Noodles, Chowmein:** Harmful ingredients are (i) salt (ii) sauce (iii) MSG (Monosodium gluconate). This chemical additive (MSG) in Chinese food is alleged to trigger migraine headache.

22. **Vada:** Harmful ingredients are salt and excess fat/oil used in frying 'Urad' dal. Otherwise it is a good source of protein because of 'urad dal' as its main constituent.

23. **Papari:** Harmful ingredients are 'maida' in fried form, salt and chutney.

24. **Pooris:** They are made from Atta (Wheat). Harmful factor in them is only the excess fat/oil used for frying them.

25. **Chopsuey:** It has the same harmful ingredients as in chowmein/noodles and it has an additional disadvantage that noodles are fried in chopsuey.

✿✿✿

Illnesses and Foods

Diet therapy in different illnesses is a big subject and deserves a complete book in itself. This chapter only touches it briefly for general guidance of readers. Readers who want to go into more details had better refer separate books pertaining to these illnesses.

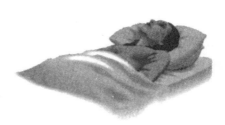

1. **Acne**
   - Cut down chocolates and sweets, highly salted snacks and extra sugar.
   - Eat plenty of shellfish, nuts etc. for zinc and fresh fruits and vegetables for vitamin C.

2. **AIDS**
   - Avoid undercooked and unwashed foods, raw or lightly cooked eggs, unpasteurised dairy products.
   - Cut down on tea, coffee, colas and alcohol.
   - Eat plenty of wholegrains, fruits and vegetables, nuts and oily fish, eggs and pasteurised dairy products.

3. **Anaemia**
   - Avoid drinking tea with meals since tannin in tea inhibits absorption of iron from food.
   - Eat plenty of fortified breakfast cereals, fresh green vegetables and fish for iron.

4. **Arthritis**
   - Cut down on highly refined foods, saturated fats, sugar and salt for osteoarthritis.

- Eat plenty of wholegrain cereals, fresh fruits and vegetables for osteoarthritis; soyabeans, tofu and fish for rheumatoid arthritis.

5. **Asthma**
   - Avoid foods that trigger attacks according to your susceptibility (e.g., foods containing additives—benzoates, sulphites or gallates; cider, wine and beer; Bread and blue cheeses; Foods, drinks and snacks containing colourings; Cow's milk, cereals, eggs, fish and nuts (especially peanuts).
   - Eat plenty of foods rich in B vitamins such as green leafy vegetables and pulses and rich in magnesium such as sunflower seeds and dried figs.

6. **Atherosclerosis**
   - Avoid smoking, physical inactivity and obesity.
   - Cut down on saturated fats, coffee and eggs.
   - Eat plenty of fruits, vegetables and oily fish.

7. **Backache**
   - Cut down on coffee, tea and other drinks containing caffeine; Fat and sugar if you are overweight; rice for reducing 'vayu' in body ('vata' dosha in ayurveda).
   - Eat plenty of cabbages, guava, papaya and kiwi fruit for vitamin C and oily fish.

8. **Bad breath**
   - Avoid garlic, onion, alcohol and all tobacco products.
   - Cut down on sugar, sweets, sweet drinks, cakes and biscuits to protect the teeth and gums and reduce plaque.
   - Take plenty of raw vegetables and apples to help to protect the gums; ginger, mustard and cinnamon (Dalchini) for the sinuses; wholegrain cereals and water to avoid constipation; carrots, broccoli, spinach and citrus fruits for beta carotene and Vit. C.

9. Blood pressure
- Avoid salty food and added salt, pickled foods, fats especially saturated fats, excessive amount of alcohol.
- Eat plenty of fresh fruits, vegetables and oily fish.

10. Bronchitis
- Avoid smoking.
- Cut down on Alcohol and caffeine.
- Eat plenty of fresh fruits and vegetables, pumpkin seeds and oily fish.

11. Cirrhosis
- Avoid Alcohol, highly spiced foods & pickles and barbequed foods.
- Cut down on fatty foods and salt.
- Eat plenty of fresh fruits and vegetables and complex carbohydrates such as potatoes, brown rice and wholegrain bread and pasta.

12. Cold
- Avoid solid foods and mucus forming foods (e.g. milk, curd, pulses such as urad, massoor, rajmah, chana, fatty and fried foods, etc.)
- Take plenty of Vit. C, garlic and onion (which act as natural decongestants), fluids to help prevent dehydration.

13. Colitis
- Avoid bran, nuts, seeds and sweetcorn.
- Eat plenty of fruits and cooked green leafy vegetables for soluble fibre, foods rich in beta carotene, oily fish for vitamin D.

14. Constipation
- Cut down on refined carbohydrates.
- Take plenty of water about 2 litres a day, take unpeeled fruits, green leafy vegetables, wholegrain cereals and wholemeal bread for insoluble fibre.

15. Cramps
- Take plenty of water before, during and after exercise to prevent dehydration, foods rich in calcium such as dairy

products and fish, nuts and seeds for magnesium, vitamin B_2 (riboflavin) from fortified breakfast cereals and yoghurt, avocados and vegetable oils for vitamin E and fish or eggs for vitamin B_{12} if the problem is night cramps.

16. Cystitis (bladder infection)

- Cut down on hot spicy foods and tea, coffee and fizzy drinks.
- Take plenty of water or other fluids and cranberry juice.

17. Diabetes

- Avoid being overweight.
- Cut down on sugary sweetened soft drinks, cakes, confectionery and chocolate; Limit salt and salty foods; Reduce alcohol intake; Cut down on fats.
- Eat regular meals; Eat more starchy & high fibre foods such as wholemeal bread, beans, peas and lentils; Eat lot of fresh fruits & vegetables for soluble fibres & vitamins but beware of very sweet fruits such as grapes or mangoes or dates; drink water or sugar free drinks.

18. Diarrhoea

- Avoid all foods (except those listed below) for the first 48 hours.

  (a) Banana (b) Water (mixed with lemon & ginger)

  (c) Boiled white rice and dry white toast

  (d) Apples   (e) Curd   (f) Khichari
- Take plenty of water to replace lost fluid, Bananas for potassium, boiled white rice for low fibre carbohydrate and apples.

Note: Alcohol & caffeine shouldn't be consumed by the person for at least 2 days after the symptoms have gone.

19. Eczema

- Avoid any foods that exacerbate or trigger your eczema such as milk and eggs. Avoid touching materials or foods known to cause contact dermatitis.

20. Emphysema

- Avoid smoking.
- Eat plenty of foods that provide vitamin C such as citrus fruits and blackcurrants; foods containing beta carotene such as carrots, apricots and spinach; foods that supply vitamin E such as wholegrain cereals and sunflower oil.

21. Epilepsy

- Avoid excessive amount of alcohol and evening primrose oil.
- Take plenty of pulses to supply vitamin B_6, zinc and magnesium; calcium-rich dairy products especially milk that has been fortified with vitamin D; rice, wholemeal bread, pineapple, blackberries and figs for manganese.

22. Eye disorders

- Eat plenty of carrots, sweet potatoes and dark green vegetables for beta carotene; Fruits and vegetables for vitamin C; Nuts, fish, wholegrains, seeds and green vegetables for their B-vitamins; Seed oils, wheatgerm and avocados for vitamin E.

23. Fatigue

- Cut down on sugar, cakes, biscuits and sweets; caffeine in tea, coffee and colas; alcohol.
- Eat plenty of iron rich foods, zinc rich foods, dark green vegetables for folate, complex carbohydrates, fish and egg for vit. B_{12}.

24. Fever

- Avoid all hard to digest foods.
- Take plenty of fluids, especially fruit juices and small light meals like khichari.

25. Flatulence

- Cut down on pulses such as peas, beans and lentils; brussels sprouts, cabbage and artichokes.
- Take plenty of yoghurt, herbs known to aid digestion, peppermint and fennel teas.

26. Fractures

- Avoid bran products, unleavened bread and brown rice.
- Eat plenty of dairy products, nuts and pulses which are good sources of calcium; oily fish for vitamin D.

27. Gallstones

- Avoid fried and fatty food and obesity.
- Eat plenty of starchy foods, such as bread and rice, fresh fruit and vegetables, oat bran and pulses for soluble fibre.

28. Gastroenteritis

- Avoid all foods (except as mentioned below) for the first 48 hours.
- Take plenty of water to replace lost fluid, Bananas for potassium, boiled white rice and dry white toast for low fibre carbohydrate, apples to cleanse the digestive system.

29. Haemorrhoids

- Avoid curries and other hot and spicy foods.
- Cut down on refined carbohydrates.
- Take plenty of apples, beans, oats, pears and cooked green leafy vegetables for their soluble fibre, wholemeal bread and brown rice for insoluble fibre and water.

30. Hair and Scalp problems

- Eat plenty of dark green leafy vegetables, carrots, sweet potatoes and egg for beta carotene and vitamin A; vegetable oils, nuts and oily fish for essential fatty acids; fish and pumpkin seeds for zinc.

31. Headache

- Cut down on excessive caffeine in coffee, strong tea and cola drinks and alcohol.
- Eat plenty of regular light meals to prevent low blood sugar levels; cold-pressed vegetable oils; avocados, nuts and seeds for vitamin E.

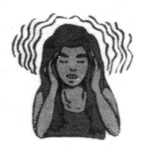

32. Immune system weakness
- Cut down on animal fats, sugar, alcohol, caffeine and highly processed carbohydrates.
- Eat plenty of protein rich foods; citrus fruits for Vit. C, vegetable oils for Vit. E, spinach, sweet potatoes and carrots which supply beta carotene.

33. Impotence
- Cut down on alcohol, coffee, tea, cola drinks and smoking.
- Eat plenty of zinc rich foods.

34. Indigestion
- Avoid heavy or fatty meals at night and smoking.
- Cut down on (i) Alcohol (ii) refined carbohydrates (iii) deep fried foods and other foods with a high fat content (iv) coffee (v) fizzy drinks.
- Eat plenty of (i) fresh fruits (ii) vegetables & vegetable juices, (iii) herbs & certain spices to improve digestion, (iv) more water (v) small frequents meals.

35. Infertility
- Cut down on alcohol, tea and highly refined foods.
- Eat plenty of (i) Citrus fruits for Vit. C (ii) Nuts, sunflower & sesame seeds & shellfish for zinc (iii) Iron rich foods (iv) Brown rice, wheatgerm, pulses, oily fish and fresh nuts for Vit. B & E. (v) Soyabeans, almonds and wholemeal bread for magnesium.

36. Influenza
- Take plenty of fluids specially diluted fruit juices, small light meals (such as khichri), garlic which has antiviral properties.

37. Insomnia
- Avoid late night meals that are greasy, spicy, rich or heavy.
- Cut down on caffeine found in coffee, tea, cola drinks and chocolate.

- Take plenty of (i) Sweetened milky malted bedtime drinks or other hot drinks with honey (ii) Starchy foods such as pasta, rice and potatoes in the evening meal.

38. Irritable Bowel Syndrome

- Avoid bran and foods that are known to produce wind such as peas, lentils and beans.
- Cut down on high fibre breakfast cereals.
- Take plenty of fresh fruits & vegetables which provide soluble fibre, live natural yoghurt and six glasses of water a day.

39. Jaundice

- Avoid alcohol.
- Cut down on spicy and fatty foods.
- Eat plenty of soyabean, egg and fish for protein, iron and B vitamins; green cabbage and pulses for folate; oats etc., which are good sources of fibre.

40. Joint problems

- Avoid obesity.
- Eat plenty of (i) Fresh fruits and vegetables for beta carotene and Vit. C (ii) Avocados, nuts and sunflower seeds for Vit. E (iii) Oily fish and shellfish for essential fatty acids (iv) Wholegrains, cereals and eggs for selenium.

41. Leukaemia

- Avoid (i) Foods which may be contaminated with bacteria or viruses such as shellfish, unpasteurised milk products and underworked meats (ii) Smoking (iii) Alcohol.
- Eat plenty of (i) Fresh fruits and vegetables for Vit. C (ii) Wholegrains, wheatgerm, molasses, nuts, pulses, fish and green leafy vegetables for B-vitamins.

42. Liver disorders

- Avoid alcohol and heavily spiced foods.

- Cut down on (i) Saturated fat from meats & dairy products (ii) Sugars (iii) Coffee and tea.
- Take plenty of (i) Foods rich in Vit. C such as citrus fruits and strawberries (ii) Vit. B_{12} found in fish and eggs (iii) Folate found in green vegetables and fruits.

43. Measles
- Avoid spicy and fried foods.
- Take plenty of (i) Fluids including diluted fruit juices (ii) Light meals including foods that supply vitamin A (iii) Fruits and vegetables that are rich in vitamin C.

44. Migraine
- Avoid (specially during attack) (i) Four 'Cs'- Chocolate, Cheese, Citrus fruits, Coffee (ii) Alcohol (iii) Garlic, onion, black grapes (iv) Tea (v) All eatables having 'tyramine' e.g., dates, bananas, spinach, eggs, broad beans, soya sauce, fig, prunes, etc. (vi) Chinese food (Monosodium gluconate (MSG) in Chinese foods often triggers migraines attack) (vii) Nitrates and Nitrites used as preservatives for some foods.
- Take plenty of (i) Regular light meals to prevent a drop in blood sugar levels (ii) Ginger in cooking or freshly grated with boiling water as a tea (iii) Magnesium rich foods.

45. Mouth Ulcers
- Avoid (i) Salt and salty foods such as chips (ii) Acidic foods such as pickles (iii) Sweets (iv) Alcohol.
- Eat plenty of (i) Dark green leafy vegetables and wholegrains for their folate (ii) Milk and potatoes for B-vitamins (iii) Foods rich in zinc such as shellfish and nuts.

46. Multiple Sclerosis
- Avoid alcohol & smoking.
- Cut down on saturated fat (dairy products & meat).
- Take plenty of (i) Wholegrains, cooked green leafy vegetables and fresh fruits for fibre and

148

energy (ii) Water to avoid constipation (iii) Poly- unsaturated fats from sunflower, safflower, corn and soya oils and oily fish.

47. Muscular Dystrophy

- Cut down on snacks between meals and high calorie foods such as cakes, biscuits and fried foods.
- Take plenty of (i) Proteins (ii) Fibre from foods such as wholemeal bread, brown rice, vegetables and fresh fruits.

48. Nail Problems

- Avoid drinks like tea which contain tannin as it inhibits iron absorption especially if taken at meal times.
- Eat plenty of (i) iron (ii) fish, pulses and nuts for zinc and selenium (iii) citrus fruit and juice for vitamin C.

49. Obesity

- Avoid (i) Full fat dairy products (ii) Fatty and sugary snacks such as biscuits, cakes, chips and nuts (iii) Nonveg foods containing high fat (iv) Alcohol.
- Eat plenty of (i) Complex carbohydrates found in pasta, potatoes, brown rice and wholegrain wheat (ii) Fresh fruit, vegetables, salads and pulses.

50. Osteoporosis

- Cut down on (i) Foods rich in phytic acid such as wheat bran, brown rice and nuts (ii) Foods containing oxalic acid such as spinach, chocolate (iii) Alcohol (iv) Salt (v) Caffeine.
- Take plenty of (i) Foods rich in calcium such as milk and dairy products (ii) Food sources of vitamin D such as oily fish and eggs (iii) Sensible exposure of skin to sunlight.

51. Palpitations
- Cut down on (i) Coffee, tea, chocolate and cola drinks which all contain caffeine (ii) Smoking (iii) Alcohol.

52. Parkinson's Disease
- Take plenty of (i) Fibre rich wholegrains, prunes, fresh fruits and vegetables to relieve constipation and to provide vitamins B, C and E (ii) Fluids at least 1.7 litres a day.

53. Peptic Ulcers
- Cut down on Salt and soya sauce, spicy foods, caffeine in coffee, tea and cola drinks, alcohol.
- Eat plenty of (i) Vegetables rich in beta carotene and fruits containing vitamin C (ii) Zinc rich food such as wholegrains.

54. Pneumonia
- Avoid smoking and polluted environment.
- Take plenty of (i) Fluids especially fruit juices (ii) Fresh fruits and vegetables (iii) Oily fish, eggs and other good sources of vitamin A.

55. Premenstrual syndrome (PMs)
- Avoid alcohol.
- Cut down on Salt & Caffeine (in tea, coffee, etc.)
- Eat plenty of (i) Small frequent meals high in carbohydrate and low in fat (ii) Foods containing Vit. B_6 such as fish and wholegrains.

56. Prostate Problems
- Cut down on tea and coffee, alcohol and dairy products.
- Eat plenty of (i) Zinc rich foods such as shellfish (ii) Foods containing Vit. E particularly wheatgerm oil, nuts, seeds and green vegetables (iii) Oily fish (e.g. herring, sardines, mackerel).

57. Sinusitis
- Eat plenty of (i) Fresh fruits and vegetables for vitamin C (ii) Shellfish and nuts for zinc (iii) Wholegrain cereals and pulses for B-Vitamins (iv) Sunflower seeds, seed oils and avocados for Vit. E (v) Garlic and onions (vi) Decongestant herbs and spices such as ginger.

58. Sore Throat

- Avoid (i) Tobacco and alcohol (ii) Chilled water and drinks.
- Take plenty of (i) Fruits & vegetables for Vit. C (ii) Foods rich in Vit. A and beta-carotene such as carrots and spinach (iii) Oily fish for Vit. D (iv) Olive oil and avocados for Vit. E (v) Yoghurt to protect against the effects of antibiotics.

59. Sunburn

- Take Plenty of (i) Water (ii) Orange coloured fruits & vegetables and dark green leafy vegetables for beta carotene and Vit. C (iii) Nuts and wheatgerm for Vit. E and zinc (iv) Wholegrains, fish and pulses for their B-vitamins.

60. Thrombosis

- Cut down on (i) Animal and dairy products which are high in saturated fats and cholesterol (ii) Salt, which raises blood pressure (iii) Smoking.
- Eat plenty of (i) Oily fish for Omega-3 fatty acids (ii) Oat bran and pulses for soluble fibre for reducing cholesterol (iii) Onion and garlic which may help to prevent blood clots.

61. Thyroid disorders

- Cut down on (i) Raw cabbage, turnips, peanuts and mustard which can inhibit the body's ability to use iodine (ii) Smoking, alcohol and caffeine if the problem is an overactive thyroid gland.

62. Tooth and gum disorders

- Avoid (i) Sweet drinks and snacks between meals (ii) Sticky foods that lodge between the teeth (iii) Regular consumption of acid drinks.
- Eat plenty of (i) Calcium rich foods such as low fat milk, yoghurt and cheese (ii) Fresh fruits and vegetables for Vit. C.

✿✿✿

Reduce 6 'S' for Healthy Living

- SUGAR & SWEETS
  - SALT
    - SPICE
      - SATURATED FATS
        - SMOKING
          - STRESS & STRAIN

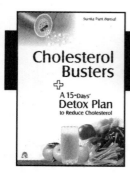

Cholesterol Busters
A 15-Days' Detox Plan to Reduce Cholesterol

—Sunita Pant Bansal

Over the past decades there has been a growing concern world over about the higher deposits of cholesterol in human body resulting in life-threatening diseases in millions of people. The solution is to understand the genesis of the problem and devise ways to be free from it.

The author opines that it is not only higher intake of fats but other factors such as excess weight, lack of exercise, alcohol, smoking and stress which lead to high level of cholesterol in human body. She further focuses on cholesterol-busting food and suggests a fifteen-days' DETOX programme yielding fantastic results in 6-8 weeks.

Pages: 104
Price: Rs. 60/- • Postage: 15/-

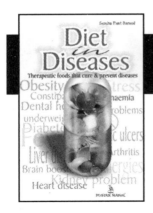

Diet in Diseases

—*Sunita Pant Bansal*

Diet plays a crucial role in promoting or preventing a disease. Especially when down with a disease, simply swallowing pills will not prove as effective if dietary guidelines are ignored. The appropriate therapeutic diet can speed up the recovery process and even boost the immune response. However, diet is one aspect of therapy that even doctors many a times fail to give due importance to. Simply put, over-nutrition, under-nutrition or wrong nutrition must equally be avoided if one wishes to stay slim, trim and fighting fit.

This book lists an array of ailments and conditions and outlines the right diet that could cure or control these problems. Once you begin having balanced, sensible meals, it won't be long before you kiss goodbye to those pills. This book will show you how to eat right and stay fit.

Demy Size • Pages: 104
Price: Rs. 69/- • Postage: Rs. 15/-

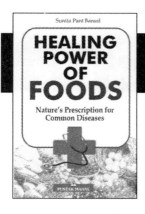

Healing Power of FOODS

—*Sunita Pant Bansal*

Nature's Prescription for Common Diseases

Hippocrates, the father of medicine, recognised that the medical therapy must be consistent with the nature and the design of the human body. He believed that the effective health care could not be separated from nutrition. He stressed prevention of disease by strongly recommending a balanced diet with a moderate and sensible lifestyle. Hippocrates wrote, "Natural forces within us are the true healers of disease... Everything in excess is opposed to nature... To do nothing is sometimes a good remedy." His philosophy was very much akin to the holistic health perspective of today.

The various foods provide not only nutrition to our body, but can prove to be medicinal too. 'Healing power of Foods' introduces all the main food groups to the reader, giving details about the medicinal uses of the commonly used foods from these groups. The tips given are simple, practical and effective. The healthy recipes at the end of the book complete the role of the various foods in providing nutritional as well as medicinal benefits.

Size: 5.5"x8.5" • Pages: 136
Price: Rs. 88/- • Postage: Rs. 15/-

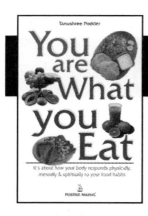

You are
What you Eat

—Tanushree Podder

It's about how your body responds physically, mentally & spiritually to your food habits

Did you know that food could heal, cure, elevate moods, improve memory, make the brain sharper, provide us with potent energy and fill us with vigour?

Food has been discovered to be the greatest natural pharmacy that is available to human beings. The right food can help us perform to our peak capacity while the wrong food can lead us towards disease and ill health.

The ordinary cabbage and cauliflower could ward off the possibility of cancer, tomatoes can effectively take care of free radicals in today's environment and carrots can provide you with the essential beta-carotene to fight off many diseases. It is surprising how effectively food can alleviate most of our common ailments.

The mysteries of the power of food and the secrets of food elements have been unravelled so that you can use food for other benefits rather than just appeasing hunger.

Demy Size • Pages: 184
Price: Rs. 96/- • Postage: Rs. 15/-

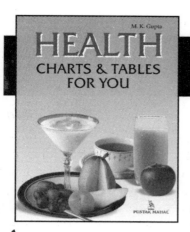

HEALTH CHARTS & Tables for You

—*M.K. Gupta*

As any health-conscious person knows, health is truly wealth. Yet, simply harbouring good intentions does not ensure good health for anyone. Beginning in infancy and right up to our twilight years, a conscious attempt has to be made to lead a healthy lifestyle. In the formative years, our parents make this effort on our behalf. But as we enter the teens and take control of our own destinies, how well informed we are on health-related issues makes all the difference between physical well-being and ill health.

This book ensures you have all the facts, figures and data at your fingertips to promote proper health and nutrition in order to prevent disease. Indeed, the cost of prevention is a pittance compared to the cost of a cure. Towards this end, *Health Charts & Tables for You* has it all: height and weight charts, blood pressure and pulse rate charts, calorie charts, fat and cholesterol charts, vitamin and mineral charts, balanced diet charts, pollution health hazard charts, infectious diseases and immunisation charts, healthy heart and stress charts... not to mention other relevant charts, tables and data.

So, if health has always been your problem, this book is just what the doctor ordered. And if health has been your forte, this book is exactly what the doctor would recommend to maintain you in the pink of your health. Either way, *Health Charts & Tables for You* is a must-read for all people.

Big Size • Pages: 144
Price: Rs. 96/- • Postage: Rs. 15/-

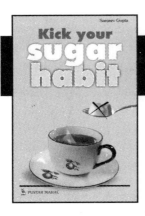

Kick Your Sugar Habit

—Sanjeev Gupta

Many of us surely do not know about sugar and its role in our life. This book shall help readers in knowing if they are sugar addicts. Once established, they can have an insight into their sugar habits and thus develop urge to control the sugar intake. This book is designed to encourage you to take control of your life and regulate health, through some crucial data that have not been available to the general public before.

Sugar eating is linked to disease. It causes some and modulates the other. It weakens our defence against illness. But to understand that you need to know all about sugar, all types of sugar, all that sugar does to our body and how, and to control that you need a few suggestions and information that constitute bulk of this effort.

This book includes:

❖ Sugar: Is there a problem? ❖ What are sugars? ❖ Sugar and health ❖ How to manage sugar habit ❖ Non-nutritive sweeteners (artificial sugars) ❖ A good diet for sugar lovers.

Demy Size • Pages: 96
Price: Rs. 68/- • Postage: Rs. 15/-

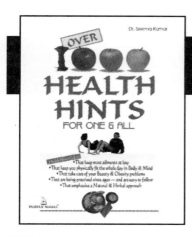

Over 1000 Health Hints
for one & all
—*Dr. Seema Kumar*

With ever-rising ground, water and atmospheric pollution, every other day, one hears the name of a new disease. Ever since man began drifting away from Nature, he is falling into the trap of a materialistic lifestyle that has desensitised him. Today, we breathe air thick with exhaust fumes, eat processed junk food that has no nutritive value, drink toxic carbonated beverages and lead sedentary lives. All of this ensures that we are plagued with different kinds of problems at regular intervals.

This book shows you how to go back to Mother Nature to beat even the most troublesome and chronic ailments. With natural preventive measures that emphasise diet, exercise and herbal remedies, there are no fears of obnoxious side effects.

Whatever be your problem – diabetes, blood pressure, asthma, acne, menopause, obesity, stomach ailments, premature ageing or general complaints – this book shows you a safe, natural and enjoyable means to overcome it. Most of the ingredients mentioned in the book are the kind available in home gardens or off the kitchen shelf.

Once you have read this book from cover to cover, you need not rush to the doctor every now and then, but will be able to take care of your own and your family's health yourself.

Big Size • Pages: 168
Price: Rs. 96/- • Postage: Rs. 15/-